Achieving Evidence-Based Practice

To my family, which grew along the way
Susan Hamer

To Mum and Dad, thanks for always being there
Gill Collinson

For Baillière Tindall

Senior commissioning editor: Jacqueline Curthoys
Project development manager: Karen Gilmour
Project manager: Jane Shanks

Achieving Evidence-Based Practice

A Handbook for Practitioners

Edited by

Susan Hamer BA MA RGN FETC(Dist) NDNCert

Programme Director,
Centre for the Development of Nursing Policy and Practice,
University of Leeds, UK

Gill Collinson RGN BSc MA Advanced Diploma in Therapeutic Counselling & Management of Change

Independent Development Consultant and Counsellor,
formerly Assistant Regional Nurse Director,
NHS Executive,
Anglia and Oxford, UK

Foreword by

Dr J A Muir Gray CBE MD FRCP(Glas&Lond)

Director,
Institute of Health Sciences,
Department of Primary Public Health,
University of Oxford, UK

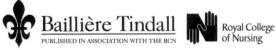

Baillière Tindall
PUBLISHED IN ASSOCIATION WITH THE RCN

Royal College
of Nursing

EDINBURGH   LONDON   NEW YORK   OXFORD   PHILADELPHIA   ST LOUIS   SYDNEY
TORONTO   1999

BAILLIÈRE TINDALL
An imprint of Elsevier Science Limited

First published 1999
  Reprinted 2000, 2003

0 7020 2349 3

British Library Cataloguing in Publication Data
A catalogue record for this book is available from the British Library

Library of Congress Cataloging in Publication Data
A catalog record for this book is available from the Library of Congress

Note
Medical knowledge is constantly changing. As new information becomes
available, changes in treatment, procedures, equipment and the use of
drugs become necessary. The editors, contributors and the publishers
have, as far as it is possible, taken care to ensure that the information
given in this text is accurate and up to date. However, readers are
strongly advised to confirm that the information, especially with regard
to drug usage, complies with the latest legislation and standards of
practice.

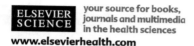 your source for books,
journals and multimedia
in the health sciences
www.elsevierhealth.com

The
publisher's
policy is to use
paper manufactured
from sustainable forests

Printed in China

Contents

Contributors

David C Benton RGN RMN BSc MPhil
Chief Executive, National Board for Nursing Midwifery and Health
Visiting for Scotland, Edinburgh, UK

Anne Brice BA DipLib ALA
Assistant Director, Health Care Libraries Unit, University of Oxford, John
Radcliffe Hospital, Oxford, UK

Stephanie Carson BSc(Hons) MBA
Consortia Performance Manager, Education and Training, NHS Executive
Northern and Yorkshire, Durham, UK

Gill Collinson RGN BSc MA Advanced Diploma in Therapeutic Counselling and Management
of Change
Independent Development Consultant and Counsellor; formerly Assistant
Regional Nurse Director, NHS Executive, Anglia and Oxford, UK

Fran Corfield RGN RSCN RHV DPSN Cert Ed(Paeds) HVL LLB(Hons) MA Cert
Adv. Practice(Mass)
Lecturer in Nursing, School of Health Care Studies, University of Leeds,
UK

Rumona Dickson MHSc BN
Coordinator, Research Synthesis, Research and Development Support
Unit, School of Health Science, University of Liverpool, UK

Gayle A Garland RGN BN MSN
Programme Director, Centre for the Development of Nursing Policy and
Practice, University of Leeds, UK

Susan Hamer BA MA RGN FETC(Dist) NDN Cert
Programme Director, Centre for the Development of Nursing Policy and
Practice, University of Leeds, UK

Debra Humphris RGN PhD MA DipN(Londs) RNT
Senior Research Fellow, Health Care Evaluation Unit, St George's
Hospital Medical School, London, UK

Lesley Joyce RN DNCert MSc Bphil
Senior Lecturer, School of Health and Community Care, Leeds
Metropolitan University, UK

Judith Palmer BSc PhD DipLib FLA
Director, Health Care Library and Information Services, University of
Oxford, John Radcliffe Hospital, Oxford, UK

Bryce Taylor MPhil DipHumPsych DipCouns. CertEd
Director: Organisation and Strategy, Oasis Human Relations, Boston Spa,
West Yorkshire, UK

Foreword

The term 'evidence-based medicine' was introduced by the group who coined it in North America not because they believed clinicians were not using science but because they believed that they were not using it explicitly, carefully and in its proper place. One of the benefits that has emerged from the focus on evidence-based decision making has been a clearer distinction between the role that evidence and values play in decision making. Formally decision-makers wandered aimlessly and unknowingly from assertions unsubstantiated by evidence to propositions supported by evidence but at least now there is a much clearer distinction between personal opinions based on values and statements based on evidence.

Furthermore, the focus on evidence, which is by and large derived from studies of groups patients, has raised much more clearly the problems of applying evidence to the individual patient. The clinician discussing and option with an individual patient has to think not only about the evidence but also about that patient's condition and that patient's values. This clearly demonstrates the way in which evidence can be best used not only in its own right but also to clarify the need to focus on the individual and their values.

The book is comprehensive and clear and will have a major impact on clinical practice in the 2^{1st} century.

Dr JA Muir Gray

Introduction

When we set out upon this journey, we were initially driven by a sense of frustration. As practitioners, we both have career pathways whose primary focus is about linking research to practice. Increasingly we have been expected, and indeed paid on occasions, to help develop colleagues' thinking in this area. All too frequently, we have sat in long meetings where resources for primary research are debated at length, and seen as the solution to providing a research-based health service. The needs of non-medical groups and whether they should be made a special case continue to engender much debate.

We met in the 1980s, a time of great change and real opportunities, which also provided us with the policy shift to press again our view that, whilst carrying out research was difficult, it represented only a small part of the equation. Equally if not more difficult was understanding and changing practice.

Ten years on we have pooled our experiences with that of colleagues in the field to produce this handbook. We hope that, through your explorations of the text, you will gain a greater understanding and share with us our awareness that no stage of achieving evidence-based practice is easy or value-free – that even by switching on a computer you commit yourself to a pathway of enquiry that has its own strengths and weaknesses. We will encourage you to reflect on your own professional behaviour and that of colleagues, and to consider whether you need to change. We do fully appreciate that changing any behaviour, whatever and wherever the evidence comes from, is complex, fun and above all a collective responsibility.

This book is intended, as the title suggests, to be a handbook, a guide to your thinking. We have structured the text to enable you to dip in and out. There are three sections. Section A is about enabling you to look for and appraise the evidence with a well informed eye. Section B considers how you would apply the evidence using a variety of approaches and in different organisational contexts. Section C is designed to enable you to understand dimensions of personal and organisational change and its ethical components.

As the world in which we work changes so rapidly we have, wherever possible, identified principles to support the ideas being promoted. The book contains lots of examples, ideas and questions. We hope you enjoy the debate.

Susan Hamer
Gill Collinson

1

Section 1

Looking for the Evidence

Evidence-based practice

Susan Hamer

KEY ISSUES

◆ Major influences in the development of evidence-based practice

◆ The stages to achieving evidence-based practice

◆ The relationship between evidence and clinical judgement

◆ Potential disadvantages associated with the evidence-based movement

◆ Evidence-based management.

INTRODUCTION

The following chapter sets out to describe evidence-based healthcare. In doing this it will consider a number of different facets. By the end of this chapter you will be able to:

- understand the major influences in the development of evidence-based healthcare
- identify key terminology
- begin to identify your development needs in relation to achieving evidence-based practice
- increase your understanding of the current limitations to achieving evidence-based practice.

EVIDENCE-BASED HEALTHCARE

The dawning of the information age has had a major impact on all our lives, and the rapidity of its development may leave us breathless at times.

It has, however, had many consequences, and the health service is not exempt. Information, and the flow of information throughout the world, has transformed the decision-making processes of practitioners. No longer do we compare our results with those of the unit next door: we are more likely to look for solutions, choices, and outcomes for patients that represent the best available knowledge internationally. It is in this world since the 1970s that the term evidence-based healthcare has become increasingly used in the UK.

The development of evidence-based healthcare has paralleled the availability of information. Technology has increased the availability of research findings and the development of research methodology. Paradoxically, because of its reliance on the power of information, this is also what makes evidence-based healthcare significant in its potential for both good and harm.

As we have noted, although evidence-based healthcare is not new, its popularity has grown. The initial debates concerning evidence-based healthcare tended to centre on research findings and their implementation, but in the late 1980s a number of factors combined and resulted in a surge of activity and interest (Box 1.1).

Box 1.1 Factors contributing to the rise in evidence-based healthcare

◆ Cost pressures

◆ Technological advances

◆ Increase in management-led decision making

◆ Consumer awareness

◆ Value for money movement

◆ Availability of information

◆ Political consensus

◆ Non-clinicians with the authority to question effectiveness

◆ International consensus

◆ Professional accountability

◆ Changing demographic profile

The context was set in which evidence-based healthcare could develop. Initially, however, much of the progress was dominated by work in the field of medicine.

EVIDENCE-BASED MEDICINE

Evidence-based medicine has been defined as 'the process of systematically finding, appraising and using contemporaneous research findings as the basis for clinical decisions' (Rosenberg and Donald, 1995, p. 1122).

The history of evidence-based medicine can be traced to the work of a group of researchers at MacMaster University in Ontario, Canada (Lockett, 1997). These researchers set out to redefine the practice of medicine so that information could be used more readily. Faced with findings that viewed medicine as being based on clinical experience rather than medical evidence, and characterised by individual bias and poor recording of results, they proposed to shift medical practice into a culture where unbiased recorded information and patient benefits were valued.

Reflections   Consider the following points in relation to your own practice:

1. Do you place a high value on accurate, unbiased, recorded information?
2. How would a member of the public know this?
3. Are patient benefits the first priority when changes to practice are being considered?

Lockett (1997) proposes the following principles as a basis for evidence-based medicine:

- Clinical experience and instincts are crucial to practising medicine. However, there is a need to record clinical experience in an unbiased and reproducible way, to enable a body of knowledge to be acquired.
- The study of pathophysiology is not a sufficient basis for understanding illness.
- Clinical information should be subject to rules of evidence to enable the diagnosis and treatment of a disease to be evaluated correctly both by the clinician and in the literature.

These principles are equally applicable to any practitioner in the health service and serve to unify our vision when trying to achieve evidence-based practice in complex organisations. Indeed, there has been much debate about whether non-medical groups of practitioners have a role to play in the evidence-based medicine movement (Kitson, 1997). Perhaps by revisiting some of the original principles, in order to anchor evidence-based medicine in its outcome, namely that of unbiased recorded information and patient benefits, we can be clearer about some of the processes subsequently adopted by organisations that have left some practitioners feeling excluded from the debate.

Kitson (1997), in a detailed analysis of the current presentation of both evidence-based medicine and clinical effectiveness, analysed the impact of three implicit assumptions on the role of non-medical groups. These assumptions are:

1. Clinicians directly involved in delivering patient care influence, either positively or negatively, patient outcomes.
2. Clinicians assume full responsibility for their practice.
3. Clinicians draw on and contribute to a body of knowledge elucidating best evidence and optimum effectiveness.

Reflections Think of your own practice and consider whether you meet these expectations. Could you provide evidence to support your view?

Kitson (1997) concluded that nursing was able to demonstrate its commitment to patient care based on meeting these assumptions, but argued that some of the limitations to the involvement of non-medical groups have been due to too narrow a focus being adopted. This was a consequence of the unidisciplinary approach used initially in the evidence-based movement. There are clearly advantages to broadening this approach out.

EVIDENCE-BASED PRACTICE

The term evidence-based practice is an amalgam of the terminology of science and professional practice: 'evidence based' implies the concepts of scientific rationality, and 'practice' is about individual practitioner behaviour (Lockett, 1997). Within its very definition lies a potential tension, a point we shall return to. As a process, evidence-based practice is about finding, appraising and applying scientific evidence to the treatment and management of healthcare (Fig. 1.1). Its ultimate goal is to support practi-

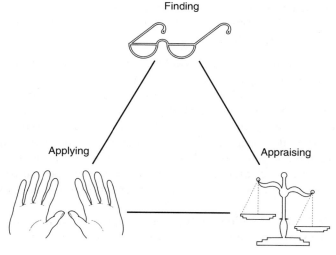

Figure 1.1 Stages of evidence-based practice.

tioners in their decision making in order to eliminate the use of ineffective, inappropriate, too expensive and potentially dangerous practices.

If we are to take action to improve the effectiveness of our health services, there are four areas that are seen as being particularly important professional considerations for moving practice forward (Walshe and Ham, 1997):

1. A scientific culture – moving away from clinicians' personal experiences and opinions and emphasising the importance of scientific enquiry.

2. Managing knowledge – the need to organise and systematise knowledge to present it intelligibly and appropriately, ensuring that it reaches the individuals or organisations that need it.

3. Systems for change – the use of formal systems such as audit for critically analysing the quality and acceptability of care. This needs to be matched by a clear understanding of what makes practitioners change their practice.

4. Incentives to perform – the need for incentives that encourage effective clinical practice and certainly do not discourage it.

Reflections Think of whether there are any disincentives to you changing your practice. Consider the impact of such issues as cash-limited budgets, block contracts and patient expectations on changes you have considered.

Strengths	Weaknesses
Practitioners confident at changing practice	Limited research data in non-medical, non-pharmacological areas
Increasingly well prepared practitioners	Patchy access to information services
Expectation of evidence-based activity in job specifications	Critical appraisal skills variable
Potential for multiprofessional working to agree outcomes collectively	Internet idiosyncratic in its development and usefulness
Reflective culture	Time
Established accountability systems	
Opportunity	**Threats**
Current policy environment	Positivistic view dominates; alternative sources of evidence not valued
Political consensus	
Management prepared to support good evidential cases in business planning processes	Patients' needs for accessible information not central to developments
Relationship between health service and university sector	Increased volume of expectations with no time for reflection
Clinical governance	

Figure 1.2 SWOT for the introduction of evidence-based practice.

Clearly, achieving evidence-based practice requires careful consideration and it may be useful to consider your own organisation's preparedness to support it. Figure 1.2 is a SWOT that we have prepared to consider its introduction in the current health service.

Reflections   If you were to do a SWOT in your own work context, what would it look like? Perhaps try this technique the next time you meet with your colleagues to consider any change in practice.

ECONOMIC EVALUATION

Most efforts to move towards evidence-based practice have focused on clinical effectiveness (does it work?) (for more information, see Ch. 5) rather than cost effectiveness (is it worth it?). Compared with clinical evaluation, economic assessment of innovative and existing interventions and services is relatively new. Most existing technologies have not been subject to the kind of economic scrutiny applied to pharmaceutical products.

Different analysis techniques can be used to answer different questions:

- Cost–benefit analysis – compares an intervention's cost and benefits using the same monetary units of measurement.
- Cost effectiveness – compares the costs of achieving a given 'effect' using different practice interventions.
- Cost utility – designed to cope with situations where there is more than one type of effect from the intervention and these need to be valued in relation to one another.
- Cost minimisation – occurs when the results of interventions are shown to be identical and a simple comparison of cost can occur.

It would seem apparent that when evidence-based change is being considered the same detailed consideration should be given to economic aspects as to clinical aspects, yet this remains difficult to achieve as the number of appropriately skilled practitioners such as health economists remains small.

APPLYING THE EVIDENCE

Although the processes for achieving evidence-based practice described may appear complex, they should become clearer as we explore them in more depth throughout the text. Suffice to say that much of the research carried out either fails to reach the public domain at all, or sits in academic journals largely unread by busy practitioners. The need to attach more energy to development and dissemination has finally been recognised, and with this recognition has come an awareness of the complexity of changing practitioner behaviours and indeed the behaviours of the organisations in which they work.

The first strategy for research in the UK National Health Service (NHS), *Research for Health* (Department of Health, 1991, p. 15), had as its aim 'that the content and delivery of care in the NHS is based on high quality research relevant to improving the health of the nation'. This brave and radical plan of action focused the health service on getting the research answers it needed for patients, not on agendas driven by personal interests or by the ambitions of university departments. In contrast to the previous scientific approach, which failed to consider the use to be made of findings, Michael Peckham (Department of Health, 1991) emphasised the importance of implementation, development and dissemination. It was a major policy shift which has had varying success (Walshe and Ham, 1997), but in Scott's (1997, p. 32) view 'research-based knowledge has come to form a central core of policy and management initiatives such as clinical audit, clinical effectiveness and patient care services'. This centrally driven policy has not changed with the new Labour government; indeed, one could see its as being strengthened in the recent policy statements, such as *A First Class Service* (Department of Health, 1998). As Salvage (1998, p. 62) notes, 'it fits in with Blairism rather well, with its recognition of stake-holders, its pluralism, its apparent downgrading of professional elitism and its emphasis on value for money'.

EVIDENCE-BASED DECISION MAKING

Evidence-based practice is based on the notion of rational decision making. However, several researchers (Tanebaum, 1994; Long and Harrison, 1997) have questioned whether or not practitioners make decisions rationally. Certainly, despite the attraction of pursuing our work of diagnosis, therapy and care on the basis of known research evidence, the limitations of evidence-based practice must be recognised. For many practitioners, not to act because the evidence is weak or non-existent is certainly not an option. Evidence can enhance clinical judgement but it cannot replace it. Equally, evidence does not ensure that the effective treatment is carried out well: monitoring is still required.

Perhaps more problematic is the potential to use a lack or limited amount of evidence as a way of justifying rationing decisions. As discussed above, cost effectiveness is not the same as cost consequences.

Reflections
- Have you experienced any difficulties in not being able to find evidence to support a clinical decision?
- What were the consequences, and how did you feel?
- Would you now present your case differently?

Box **1.2** A range of dissemination interventions

◆ Advice from respected colleagues

◆ Academic paper or publication

◆ Audit and feedback

◆ Clinical guidelines

◆ Conferences

◆ Workshops

◆ Outreach visits

◆ Patient-mediated interventions

◆ Reminder systems (manual or computerised)

◆ Marketing

◆ Computerised decision support systems

◆ Financial incentives

◆ Influencing curriculum content

◆ Commissioning standards

Changing practice can be more difficult than it at first seems. The field of behaviour change among health professionals is itself developing an evidence base, through which it is clear that multifaceted strategies are needed, using a range of techniques (Oxman *et al.*, 1995). A number of these are listed in Box 1.2.

Reflections   Clinical governance is expected to address how good practice can be recognised in one area and transferred to another (Scally and Donaldson, 1998). Consider an innovation you would wish to share. What techniques could you use?

EVIDENCE-BASED MANAGEMENT

Many of us have had the experience of a management decision that has had a significant impact on care outcomes yet no consultation appears to have taken place.

Reflections
- Has any management action across your organisation affected the effectiveness of your care?
- Would piloting have helped to avoid some of the problems?

As Hewison (1997, p. 196) noted, 'whilst managers and policy makers feel it is part of their role to request evidence to inform decisions and make judgements about the allocation of resources, managerial activity is not generally subject to the same expectation'. Hewison (1997) proposed that both management and clinical care have a weak evidence base and that, just as evidence-based decision making is a goal for practitioners, it should be a goal for all policy-makers too. New policy proposals should be subject to the same kind of scrutiny we demand of new clinical interventions. Organisational restructuring, the introduction of new work practices, the configuration of buildings ought all to be treated to the same decision-making rigour. Evidence-based management should be a shared goal and research resources used to support its development.

CRITICAL AWARENESS

There are many other areas in which management has a critical role to play, particularly in providing a supportive environment to the activity of evidence-based practice. This will be discussed in Chapter 9; however, in relation to developing and fostering critical awareness among practitioners (for a definition see Box 1.3), a dominant management style that fosters the following is very valuable as it:

Box 1.3 What is critical awareness?

To be critical is defined as being discerning, capable of expressing a judicious opinion and capable of reasoned judgement. However, when we refer to critical awareness we probably mean more than this. For example:

- to be questioning
- to see more than one side of an argument
- to be objective rather than subjective
- to weigh evidence
- to judge others' statements as being based on reason, evidence or logic on the one hand or based on partial evidence, special pleading, emotion or self-interest on the other
- to look at the meaning behind the facts
- to identify issues arising from the facts
- to recognise when further evidence is needed.

- encourages a problem-solving approach
- values debate and discussion
- encourages people's ideas
- values creativity and innovation
- is supportive during change
- discourages negative criticism
- values people for their contribution.

CONCLUSION

Finally, as we have already noted, the adoption of evidence-based practice means that evidence referred to is commonly located in a positivist perspective of the nature of knowledge. This sees the clinical trial as characterising a level of objectivity that all other methods should try to achieve; it is concerned with what can be measured, touched and enumerated. However, this point of view could also potentially place little value on attitudes, experiences and feelings.

Consequently any debate of evidence-based practice needs to acknowledge that the dominance of any form of research method could lead to the exclusion of information that is vital to decision-making processes. Although bounded in the language of technology, the new paradigm of evidence-based practice places more emphasis on individual practitioners; it relies on our ability to focus evidence at practice level to produce enhanced patient outcomes.

REFERENCES

Department of Health (1991). *Research for Health, A Research and Development Strategy for the NHS*. London: HMSO.
Department of Health (1998). *A First Class Service, Quality in the New NHS*. London: HMSO.
Hewison, A. (1997). Evidence based medicine, what about Evidence based management? *Journal of Nursing Management*, **5**, 195–198.
Kitson, A. (1997). Using evidence to demonstrate the value of nursing. *Nursing Standards*, **11**, 34–39.
Lockett, T. (1997). Traces of evidence. *Healthcare Today*, **July/August**, 16.
Long, A. & Harrison, S. (1997). The balance of evidence. Evidence based decision making. *Health Service Journal*, **106**, 1–2.
Oxman, A.D., Thomas, M.A., Davis, D.A. & Hayes, R.B. (1995). No magic bullets: a systematic review of 100 trials of interventions to help health professionals deliver services more effectively and efficiently. *Canadian Medical Association Journal*, **153**, 1423–1431.
Rosenberg, W. & Donald, A. (1995). Evidence based medicine, an approach to clinical problem solving. *British Medical Journal*, **310**, 1122–1126.
Salvage, J. (1998). Evidence based practice: a mixture of motives? *Nursing Times*, **94**, 61–64.
Scally, G. & Donaldson, L.J. (1998). Clinical governance and the drive for quality improvement in the new NHS in England. *British Medical Journal*, **317**, 61–65.
Scott, E. (1997). Research and development in nursing. *Nursing Times*, **93**, 32–33.
Tanebaum, S.J. (1994). Knowing and acting in medical practice: the epistemological politics of outcomes research. *Journal of Health Politics, Policy and Law*, **19**, 27–44.
Walshe, K & Ham, C. (1997). *Acting on the Evidence, Progress in the NHS*. Birmingham: NHS Confederation & University of Birmingham Health Services Management Centre.

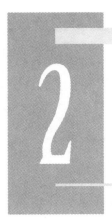

Types of evidence

Debra Humphris

INTRODUCTION

The term 'evidence' has become much used within healthcare over the past 5 years with the appearance of 'evidence-based medicine' and, more appropriately, 'evidence-based healthcare'. The term 'evidence-based' implies the use and application of research evidence as a basis upon which to make healthcare decisions, as opposed to decisions not based on evidence. Two underlying assumptions are, first that, there is research evidence and, second, that it is possible to make a judgement about its quality and usefulness. The aim of this chapter is to explore the different types of evidence that are available to you and how you can make judgements about its quality and usefulness, as you build your ability to become a discerning consumer of evidence. The key issues that will be explored will be not only the differing forms of evidence, but also the critical questions you need to think through when making judgements about evidence. As you work through the chapter you will come across a number of reflective activities; these are designed to encourage you to consider how you are questioning the evidence you encounter.

The objectives of this chapter are:

• to explore the different forms of evidence that are available
• to identify how you can make judgements about the quality and usefulness of evidence

- to explore the concept of 'generalisability' in relation to research evidence.

EVIDENCE, EVIDENCE EVERYWHERE

While the volume of research evidence expands (Williamson *et al.*, 1989; MacGuire, 1990), the scarcity of credible evidence compounds the difficulty faced by clinicians when attempting to make decisions about which evidence to use (Greer, 1988). Much of the evidence produced by researchers may not be 'practice-ready' (Brett, 1987) or clinically useful; it may need to be 'repackaged' (Kanouse and Jacoby, 1988), and its significance and usefulness to practice determined (Bircumshaw, 1990). To do this requires skills in the identification, analysis, synthesis and presentation of evidence (Haynes *et al.*, 1995) which may be beyond the scope of many individual clinicians (Eddy, 1988; Roberts *et al.*, 1995). In many cases it is here that the role of libraries and information technology has taken on growing importance (Freemantle and Watt, 1994; Weed, 1997). Throughout this chapter a range of questions will be raised that you should reasonably ask when you are critically appraising particular forms of research evidence.

Reflection   You might find it useful before you read on to list questions you think would be useful to ask of research evidence. Do your questions differ depending on the form of research evidence?

WHAT IS EVIDENCE?

We all use and interpret a wide range of sources of evidence to inform our judgements and the way we practise. That evidence may be highly variable, from our own experience to a trusted colleague's professional opinion or a randomised controlled trial you read about in a professional journal. You may take as evidence that which you were taught in your formal education (Turner and Allan Whitfield, 1997), or the word of an influential colleague. No matter which forms of evidence you draw upon they will comprise a rich and highly varied mix of sources. Therefore, as a consumer of evidence, and indeed as a generator, translator or purveyor, what becomes important is that you are able to be a discerning consumer of that evidence. You should be able to make a judgement about recognising the good from the bad, to know the strengths and weaknesses of how that evidence was generated, to appraise and utilise it critically, if appropriate, not just to take all evidence on absolute trust.

Throughout the chapter Evidence Examples are used to illustrate the range of research methods discussed. The examples will be in the form of abstracts that you would find when you are searching the literature. Each of the studies will in its way inform practice, but what you need to be able to do is to discern the *quality* of the evidence.

Evidence derived from a process of systematic research provides a basis for belief; it seeks to generate, prove or disprove a hypothesis; and it makes evident or demonstrates the basis of that proof. The nature of such proof in healthcare can lead to (Muir Gray, 1997, p. 69):

1. *that which increases the understanding of health, ill health and the process of healthcare*
2. *that which enables an assessment of the interventions used in order to try to promote health, to prevent ill health or to improve the process of healthcare*

The process by which research evidence is generated has well established methods and limitations. The transparency and clarity of that production process should enable you to make a judgement about its use in your practice. In many areas, the nature of the research question requires that a particular research methodology be employed. For example, a randomised controlled trial can examine the effectiveness of a new intervention, but a qualitative methodology will be required to understand patients' feelings about the effects of an intervention. There are also traditions of evidence and values placed upon those differing approaches, often influenced by the researcher's professional background or the wider dominance of the natural sciences, and that of positivist philosophy within medical research. Gradually there is an acknowledgement that a range of forms of research evidence helps to aid our understanding of issues, representing a form of continuum in terms of its generation (Box 2.1).

Research has been defined as 'an attempt to increase available knowledge, by discovery of new facts or relationships through systematic enquiry' (Macleod Clarke and Hockey, 1989, p. 4).

Underpinning the nature of that 'systematic scientific enquiry' is a philosophical approach or paradigm. The two major philosophical traditions in research stem from differing beliefs about the nature of truth (Fig. 2.1). Positivist, empirical science is derived from the approach of natural sciences, which is focused on the testing of a hypothesis through objective observation and validation. Such quantitative methodologies seek positive proof of associations and causal relationships and thus may

Box **2.1** A continuum of evidence					
Qualitative					**Quantitative**
Opinion based on experience	Descriptive studies	Surveys	Cohort studies	Non-randomised trials	Randomised controlled trials

Phenomenology	Positivism
Based in the social sciences, interpretative in nature Assumes social world is socially constructed Exploratory, hypothesis-generating Concerned with meanings and values Addresses questions from participants' perspectives	Based in the natural science Concerned with external reality Hypothesis testing Based on objective observation and measurement Addresses questions by measuring and describing Attempts to establish statistically significant relationships Concerned with correlation and causality
Qualitative methods: in-depth interviews, case studies, (non)participant observation, focus groups, ethnography	**Quantitative methods:** randomised controlled studies, case-controlled studies, cohort studies, surveys, statistical analysis, database analysis

Figure 2.1 Paradigms of inquiry.

have a greater degree of certainty and the generalisability of their findings (Kendall, 1997). The phenomenological approach to the generation of evidence is concerned with gaining insight into individuals' subjective experience and realities, enabling the development of theories to interpret and understand subjective experience. Qualitative methods are interpretative and found mainly in the social sciences (Kendall, 1997).

These paradigms have been developed and used with a differing emphasis in different professional groups. There is, however, a growing acknowledgement of the worth of combining methods and the need for more multimethod studies (Goodwin and Goodwin, 1984; Mishel, 1987).

No matter what research methodology is employed, all evidence has its strengths and weaknesses; the perfect piece of research has yet to be published, and from all research there are still lessons to be learned. The nature of evidence that informs practice is highly varied and not all methods are appropriate to the questions asked. The central questions to ask of all research therefore relate to the use of the appropriate method for the question, which is then conducted with transparency and robustness.

Reflection Go back to your earlier list. Would you change it at all to accommodate the different research methodologies?

It all takes time

Research evidence as a whole has some built-in constraints, such as the time lag between its generation and publication, let alone its use. As an experienced ward sister embarking on her early work on pressure sores, Doreen Norton later reflected that 'the sad thing is that much of the critical information existed in research long gone before…the fact remains, such information has not percolated through to nursing practice and teaching' (Norton, 1988).

The act of publication also introduces bias affects into research. The persons who decide what gets published in journals also make judgements about what does not get published. Journals prefer to publish research that shows an effect, and so negative or ambivalent findings may not be so attractive to an editor. Figure 2.2 attempts to illustrate that the volume of published research is only a proportion of the total research activity.

Journals also have a hierarchy, and researchers driven by the need to publish will tend to seek publication in the more 'prestigious' journals. The pressures upon researchers to publish were reflected by Brookes (1997, p. 46) who commented that:

> As long as journals continue to pursue their current editorial policies then we are restricting our view of a broader scientific picture. More worrying, though, if statistical significance increases the chance of a researcher's work being published, might not he or she be tempted to tamper a little with the data? After all, a career might depend upon it.

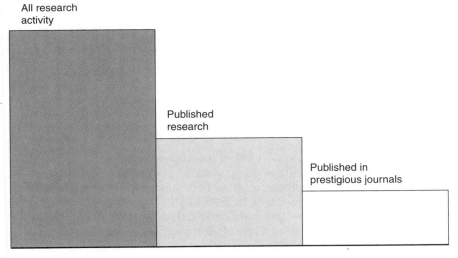

Figure 2.2 The publication of research findings.

LEVELS OF EVIDENCE

The different forms of evidence have been characterised in a hierarchy, or continuum, based on the methodology used to generate them. As you will see, the hierarchy below places greatest emphasis on evidence derived from a positivistic approach to science: the randomised controlled trial is viewed as a 'gold standard'. However, not all of these methods are appropriate for all situations, as it may indeed not be possible to collect evidence using a randomised controlled trial.

As a discerning consumer of research evidence, the questions you need to ask yourself are about the rigour of the process by which the evidence was generated that you propose to use. Remember that this chapter does not provide an exhaustive list of approaches to research generation, but should give you an idea about the relative advantages, disadvantages and appropriate use of a range of common types of methods used to generate evidence. The National Health Service (NHS) Funded Centre for Reviews and Dissemination (CRD), which undertakes systematic reviews of research, has set out what it identifies as a hierarchy of evidence (Box 2.2). This enables the Centre to be transparent about the research evidence it uses to construct a review (see Chapter 3). As you will see, this hierarchy is oriented towards positivistic forms of evidence, such as the randomised controlled trial.

Box 2.2 Hierarchies of evidence

(Clinical trials)
I   Well-designed randomised controlled trials
II-1a Well-designed controlled trials with pseudo-randomisation
II-1b Well-designed controlled trials with no randomisation

(Cohort studies)
II-2a Well-designed cohort (prospective) study with concurrent controls
II-2b Well-designed cohort (prospective) study with historical controls
II-2c Well-designed cohort (retrospective) study with concurrent controls
II-3   Well-designed case-controlled (retrospective) study
III   Large differences from comparisons between times and/or places with or without intervention (in some circumstances these may be equivalent to level I/II)
IV   Opinions of respected authorities based on clinical experience; descriptive studies and reports from expert committees

University of York, NHS Centre for Reviews and Dissemination. *Undertaking systematic reviews of research on effectiveness: CRD Guidelines for those carrying out or commissioning reviews.*

FORMS OF EVIDENCE

All research evidence is susceptible to variation and not all research is equal: the domination of the positivist, natural science paradigm as embodied in the medical sciences has placed it in a stronger position. Therefore, to consider the appropriateness of different forms of evidence, the following research designs will be used as examples:

- randomised controlled trials
- case-controlled study
- cohort study
- survey
- qualitative studies
- professional consensus.

Reflection   From the list you wrote earlier, which of these methods did you have in mind? Would you add any more questions to your list at this stage? Perhaps it is necessary to understand the mechanics of the method before you can think clearly about the questions you need to ask.

In recent years the NHS Research and Development Programme has supported two important centres of evidence collation, where certain forms of evidence are synthesised to produce systemic reviews and meta-analyses. The UK Cochrane Centre and the NHS Centre for Reviews and Dissemination are both funded as part of the NHS Research and Development Programme.

The UK Cochrane Centre and Collaboration was established in Oxford in 1992; it undertakes the meta-analysis of randomised controlled trials. The Collaboration is a global community whose role is 'to collaborate with others to build, maintain and disseminate a database of systematic, up-to-date reviews of randomised controlled trials of health care' (Sheldon and Chalmers, 1994).

The NHS Centre for Reviews and Dissemination is based at the University of York; it undertakes and coordinates systematic reviews of the literature. The reviews are on specific questions of importance to the NHS, principally in areas of effectiveness and cost-effectiveness of healthcare interventions, management and organisation of health services. The Centre also has a role in disseminating the results of its reviews to the wider community, in forms such as the Effective Health Care Bulletins, as well as maintaining a database of reviews.

These are both important centres, which in many respects act to find, filter and collate research published on specific issues and to provide it in a form that is useful to the NHS and wider communities.

RANDOMISED CONTROLLED TRIALS

Randomised controlled trials (RCTs) are often termed as the 'gold standard' in research evidence, which assumes that that standard is judged against on a positivistic scale. RCTs are the best way of evaluating an intervention, of examining a possible cause–effect relationship between variables, or comparing differing interventions. In the Evidence Example described in Box 2.3, a randomised trial compared two types of wound dressing for ease of application and removal, adhesion, conformability, absorbency and wear time. Individuals who met the criteria for the study, and consented to participate, were randomly allocated to one of two groups in each of the five study sites. Trials can also be 'blinded', the participants may be 'blinded' (i.e. they do not know which group they are in), or the whole study may be 'double blind' (the clinicians also would not know to which group an individual had been allocated). The reason for these stages in the research process is to minimise the bias of confounding factors such as the clinicians or participants behaving differently. In the Evidence Example it would have been difficult to have 'blinded' the intervention, as it would have been evident which dressing had been applied.

The RCT is an experimental design that seeks to manipulate a variable within the trial, with a group used as a control for which that variable is not manipulated. Researchers undertaking analysis of the data identify participants only by a code. The purpose of having both a control group and blinding a study is to minimise the element of bias in a study, thus seeking to ensure that any effects observed are due to the intervention.

The likely size of that effect, for example wound healing, will influence the sample size of that trial. The smaller the effect, the greater the number of people needed for the trial if it is to have sufficient statistical power to detect a change. This is a particular problem in circumstances when there may be only a small number of cases, for example rare conditions (Muir Gray, 1997).

In recent times the development of meta-analysis (i.e. the statistical aggregation of similar RCTs) has attempted to add to the power of study outcomes by increasing the total numbers included. RCTs are, therefore, dependent upon sufficient recruitment to both the control and study groups. Loss of participants can place in jeopardy or invalidate a study. A growing issue in the design of RCTs has been the need to address patient preferences in order to maintain the motivation of participants to take part in the study (Muir Gray, 1997). In the Evidence Example the loss of participants due to changes in location of care or death illustrated the difficulties of undertaking research on such a population.

In making a judgement about the quality of an RCT there are numerous checklists available; two important key points made by Pocock (1983) relate to principal and common deficiencies of trials. Principal deficiencies include:

- inadequate definition of eligible patients
- inadequate definition of treatment schedules
- inadequate definition of methods of evaluation

- lack of appropriate control group
- failure to randomise patients to alternative treatments
- lack of objectivity in patient evaluation
- failure to use blinding techniques, when appropriate.

Common deficiencies consist of:

- too few patients
- failure to account for all patients
- inappropriate statistical methods
- confusing presentation of results
- data dredging.

The RCT is viewed by some as a gold standard in terms of evidence as it attempts to reduce bias, manipulate a specific intervention and often requires study groups which are sufficiently large to demonstrate a power of effect of the intervention. However, while the unit of knowledge produced may be generalisable, it is limited by the condition and constraints upon the trial. The trial in Box 2.3 compared only two dressings and the performance of the dressings has to also be placed in the context of the case mix of the participant group.

Systematic bias may be built into the study in a number of ways: (1) selection bias in terms of the differences between the treatment and control groups; (2) bias in the way care is delivered to the intervention group or data are collected; and (3) exclusions from the trial may differ across the groups. The assessment of outcome should not differ across the groups as this would build in systematic detection bias. For a RCT to be generalisable, it must be large enough to demonstrate sufficient power of that specific intervention.

Evidence Example: Randomised controlled trial

Box **2.3** Comparison of two dressings in pressure sore management

This study compared a polyurethane foam dressing with a hydrocolloid dressing for ease of application and removal, adhesion, conformability, absorbency and wear time.

Study design   A randomised trial was carried out on 61 patients with stage II or III pressure sores in five centres in the UK. The study was designed as a randomised prospective comparison of two dressings; 61 subjects were recruited in five centres, according to the following criteria:

Box **2.3** Cont'd

- Patients aged 18 years and over who were not pregnant and who were able to understand and consent to the trial.
- Patients with no history of poor compliance in their previous involvement in the study.
- Patients with a stage II or III pressure sore (Stirling classification), with the largest diameter less than or equal to 11 cm and with no sign of infection.
- Patients allocated to one of two treatment groups sequentially for each centre using an open randomised list.

Methods   Dressings were applied for up to 30 days and assessments were carried out at each dressing change. Dressings were carried out in accordance with manufacturer's instructions and dressing performance was assessed at each change. Consistency of approach in the various centres was assured by researcher visits and regular contact with staff. Patients were entered into the study until the wound healed, or for a maximum of 30 days.

Results   Sixty patients were included in the statistical analysis; one patient was excluded because of death shortly after the first dressing application. Wounds healed in 12 patients during the trial. While the treatment groups were well matched with respect to patients and wounds, despite randomisation of patients at each centre there was an imbalance in the size of wounds treated in the two groups. Wounds treated with the hydrocolloid dressing were larger than those in the group dressed with the polyurethane foam. Forty of the 61 patients enrolled in the study were withdrawn, mainly because they were discharged before the wound healed. In order to collect more meaningful data, further studies must include larger numbers of patients to make allowance for such a high drop-out rate.

Source: Bale *et al.* (1997).

The trial method was an appropriate method for assessing the effects of the different dressings. However, the data can tell us nothing about how the participants felt about their situation, or the outcome of their wound care, or what happened to them after the trial.

Questions to ask of randomised controlled trials

To help you critically appraise this form of evidence, try using the following questions as a framework. You may find it helpful to find a similar study and read it with these questions at hand. At the same time consider the list of questions you have started constructing to see how many points you have already covered.

General questions

- Are the results of the trial valid?
- Did the trial address a clearly focused issue?
- Was the study focused in terms of:
  - the population studied?
  - the intervention given?
  - the outcome considered?
- Was the assignment of patients to the treatment randomised?
- Were all patients who entered the trial properly accounted for in its conclusions?
- Was follow-up complete?
- Were patients analysed in the groups to which they were randomised?

Source: Milne (1997).

Detail questions

- Were patients, health workers and study personnel blind to the treatment?
- Were the groups similar at the start of the study in terms of other factors that might have affected the outcome such as age, sex and social class?
- Apart from the experimental intervention, were the groups treated equally?

Analysis of the results

- How large were the treatment effects?
- What outcomes were measured?
- How precise was the estimate of treatment effect?
- What were the confidence intervals?
- What was the attrition rate and how were the data analysed?

CASE-CONTROLLED STUDIES

A case-controlled design is appropriate to use when attempting to identify cause of disease (e.g. infection diseases) or rare effects of treatment (e.g. side-effects of drug therapy). It is an inappropriate design when attempting to evaluate the effectiveness of an intervention, when a RCT is appropriate.

Participants are recruited who have the condition or diagnosis that is the subject of the study. A control group is also recruited which would comprise participants who are free of the disease, but matched to the study group in all other respects, so allowing a comparison between the two groups. As with RCTs there remains the risk of bias in terms of group selection and measurement.

In the Evidence Example in Box 2.4, a group of patients with wound infection was matched with similar surgical patients without wound infections. It was then possible to compare the two groups in respect of the variables that were suspected to have led to the complication: operative risk, procedure duration, technique in theatre, preoperative preparation.

In the Evidence Example five patients had to be excluded due to data deficiencies. This illustrates the dependence that this method has on retrospective data, such as patient records, and the range of confounding variables this can introduce. Invariably in case-controlled studies, there are some individuals in the study group to whom some outcome has already occurred, and much skill is needed in terms of matching the control group of individuals to whom that particular outcome has not occurred (St Leger, 1992).

The assumption behind a case-controlled study is that by looking retrospectively, and with skilled matching of the control group, it may be possible to identify the cause–effect relationship that may have existed, but not possible to prove it. Within a case-controlled study it is extremely important, and often very difficult, to minimise bias, decisions about selection and recruitment of individuals to both groups of the study, which can bring with it its own bias. Whilst this design may be cheaper and quicker than an RCT, it still requires sufficient numbers and sufficient data that are statistically robust, in order make appropriate comparisons.

This form of study also can infer a cause–effect relationship, but is not sufficient to confer such a relationship. As with RCTs, case-controlled studies are also dependent on maintaining sufficient numbers within both groups and there is bias associated with recruitment to those groups and retrospective documented evidence (Carter, 1996).

Evidence Example: Case-controlled study

Box **2.4** Effect of surgical would infection on postoperative hospital stay

Objective To determine the effect of surgical wound infection on postoperative duration of hospital stay.

Design A case-controlled study nested within a cohort.

Setting A tertiary care hospital.

Box 2.4 Cont'd

Patients Selected from a cohort of 4702 inpatients who underwent surgical procedures over a 12-month period. There were 3602 patients, 1100 having been excluded because of lack of infection associated with a particular surgical procedure, because of 'lumping' of procedures under a non-homogeneous heading, or because a procedure was unlikely to be the reason for the patient's hospitalisation.

Main outcome measure Postoperative duration of hospital stay.

Results In the cohort, 89 wound infections were identified, 73 of these occurring with procedures selected for study. Five patients were excluded from the study because of data deficiencies, leaving 68 patients who underwent 15 different procedures. These were compared with 136 control patients selected by stratified random sample from a list of patients who underwent the same risk-indexed procedure in the same surgical division. Patients with wound infection and controls did not differ in anaesthetic risk score or procedure duration. Patients with infection remained in hospital 19.5 days longer than controls (95% confidence interval 11.0–27.9 days). Deep-seated infection prolonged the hospital stay more than superficial incisional infection (24.3 versus 13.2 days).

Conclusion Surgical wound infection markedly prolonged the duration of hospitalisation in University of Alberta hospitals, longer than that documented in previous studies in other countries. Maximising opportunities to prevent wound infection would be beneficial to both patients and hospitals.

Source: Taylor *et al.* (1995).

Questions to ask of case-controlled studies

Here again is a framework of questions to help you appraise this form of evidence critically. From your own list, how many of these have already been covered?

- Was the aim of the study made clear?
- Were the inclusion and exclusion criteria for the sample made clear?
- How were cases recruited and what were the matching criteria?
- How was the control group recruited and what criteria were used?
- How was exposure to the independent variables measured?
- What analysis was undertaken?

Reflection   You may begin to see a number of questions that may reasonably be asked of all forms of research evidence. Can you identify these from your own list?

COHORT STUDIES

Cohort studies, as they suggest, take groups or cohorts of individuals and study them over a period of time. Cohort studies can be retrospective or prospective. Prospective studies allow the identification of data that will be collected in advance, ensuring that those data can be collected from that particular cohort. In a retrospective cohort study a group of participants, such as patients who have developed cancer or individuals who have developed diabetes over the past 20 years, forms the cohort. Retrospective studies are dependent on recall and case notes.

The cohort study is an appropriate design for identifying uncommon or adverse effects of treatments, or for assessing different approaches or changes in service delivery, management or organisation (e.g. the intro-duction of professional education changes). The cohort study design can be used to establish causation of a disease, or to evaluate the outcome of treatment, when a RCT is not possible. A cohort (population or sample of population) free of disease is selected and categorised for exposure or non-exposure to risk factors. There is then follow-up and comparison of 'exposed' and 'non-exposed' groups to test the hypothesis on causality. This may be prospective (select now, follow over time) or retrospective (where good available data exist). Retrospective studies are inexpensive and quick to carry out compared with prospective studies.

Cohort studies are often used to attempt to establish causation, usually around disease. They are particularly appropriate when evaluating the impact of treatment, especially when a RCT would not be possible. In the Evidence Example described in Box 2.5, a cohort of 143 patients was followed over a period of 6 months. Cohort studies are useful in the study of 'natural experiments' (Muir Gray, 1997). Natural experiments are situations in which changes in healthcare occur for a range of political or managerial reasons, but not in a way that can be controlled for, as in a RCT. Changes in the organisation and delivery of healthcare can be followed through with a cohort of patients or staff or hospitals, enabling the assess-ment of various approaches or changes.

It would not be possible in such a situation to say that any one approach or change was better than any other; to do that would require a RCT. However, a cohort study can provide data that could identify adverse effects or uncommon consequences of such changes. Again the issue of recruitment of participants is extremely important. Have all the people within a defined period of time or within a defined cohort been selected? (Muir Gray, 1997). Any reason for excluding people from a cohort should be viewed with suspicion: it could result in the cohort becoming unrepresentative , if the cohort is of individuals at risk or exposed to a particular disease or intervention.

In the analysis of results it is also imperative to take into account any pre-existing conditions that may have had an effect on a particular individual's outcome in relation to the study. Across the cohort there may be a severity of effect depending on the exposure, change or modification that is under study, and means must be found within the study or made explicit in the study of how this differing severity has been analysed. Cohort studies are open to abuse, the biggest abuse being the attempt to assess the effectiveness of an intervention where a RCT would be more appropriate (Muir Gray, 1997).

Evidence Example: Cohort study

Box **2.5** Role of patient's view of their illness in predicting return to work and functioning after myocardial infarction: a longitudinal study

Objective   To examine whether patients' initial perceptions of myocardial infarction predict subsequent attendance at a cardiac rehabilitation course, return to work, disability and sexual dysfunction.

Design Patients' perceptions of their illness were measured at admission with their first myocardial infarction and at follow-up 3 and 6 months later.

Setting Two large teaching hospitals in Auckland, New Zealand.

Subjects A total of 143 consecutive patients aged under 65 years with their first myocardial infarction.

Main outcome measures Attendees at rehabilitation course; time before returning to work; measures of disability with sickness impact profile questionnaire for sleep and rest, social interaction, recreational activity, and home management; and sexual dysfunction.

Results Attendance at the rehabilitation course was significantly related to a stronger belief during admission that the illness could be cured or controlled ($t = -2.08$, $P = 0.04$). Return to work within 6 weeks was significantly predicted by the perception that the illness would last a short time ($t = -2.52$, $P = 0.01$) and have less grave consequences for the patient ($t = -2.87$, $P = 0.115$). Patients' belief that heart disease would have serious consequences was significantly

Box 2.5 Cont'd

related to later disability in work around the house, recreational activities and social interaction. A strong illness identity was significantly related to greater sexual dysfunction at both 3 and 6 months.

Conclusion Patients' initial perceptions of illness are important determinants of different aspects of recovery after myocardial infarction. Specific illness perceptions need to be identified at an early stage as a basis for optimising outcomes from rehabilitation programmes.

Source: Petrie *et al.* (1996).

Questions to ask of a cohort study

To appraise this form of study design critically, you will need assurances about how the evidence was constructed. Here the issue of whether a study is concurrent or historical adds another dimension. Try using the following framework of questions:

- Was the hypothesis made clear?
- Were the inclusion and exclusion criteria for the cohort made clear?
- How was the cohort recruited?
- Were the controls historical or concurrent?
- Are the diagnostic criteria made clear?
- What measures were used?
- Were the measurement tools of known validity?

SURVEYS

The survey is one of the most commonly used methods in social science research. Surveys may use a range of instruments, questionnaires, in-depth interviews and observation (da Vaus, 1993). They provide us with information about a snapshot in time or over a period, for example a survey of hospital waiting lists at the end of a financial year. Surveys can collect a range of types of data from opinions to quantifiable facts (Muir Gray, 1997), through which it is possible to collect sufficient data about the variables under study to undertake analysis or to explore associations and correlations.

Depending on the purpose of a study, care and attention must be paid to sample size and the population from which the data are collected. If, as in the case of the General Household Survey, which occurs once a decade, the population is the entire population, this is referred to as a census. More often, however, surveys attempt to gather data from a sample of the population which should be sufficiently large to be representative of the defined population.

Sampling may be undertaken by means of a simple random sample, but how the sampling frame is defined should be made evident. The Evidence Example in Box 2.6 states that it used a 'convenient sample': this is a non-probability sample, often comprising participants who are readily available. In the case of a survey utilising a questionnaire, it should be made clear the process by which the questionnaire was generated or whether an existing instrument of known validity and reliability has been used.

The structure of questionnaires is also extremely complex; they need to be developed and tested, and be suitable for collecting the data required. Questionnaires, typically, do not allow the researchers to go back to the participants from whom they collected the data to clarify information (da Vaus, 1993). The wording, construction, format, layout and method of administration of questionnaires are all capable of influencing and biasing the study and its response rate.

Reflection   Wording questions to ensure that they are not misunderstood is not as easy as it may seem. Try to write a question that would ask participants about their academic level of qualifications. You are unable to go back to the participants to ask for clarification, so you have to get it right the first time. When you have written your question, try it out on some friends.

Surveys can be completed face to face, such as in a market survey, via telephone interviews or directly through the post. For all of these techniques there are clear advantages and disadvantages. Whichever method is adopted, the resources available will influence the decision, the nature of access to the population, the amount of money, time and size of study required (da Vaus, 1993). In each case, what is important is that researchers make clear the known limitations and methods used within their study and their appropriateness to the particular situation or question they are attempting to answer.

Non-response bias also needs to be considered. In the Evidence Example given in Box 2.6 from the UK data, 140 participants (44%) did not respond; therefore the survey does not have data on just under half the possible respondents. The researchers are left not knowing why these individuals did not respond, or what their responses might have been.

Evidence Example: Survey

Box **2.6** Use of evidence-based practice in physiotherapy: a cross-national study

This study investigated clinical physiotherapists' reasons for treatment techniques with a particular focus on the utilisation of

Box **2.6** Cont'd

journal review and research literature. Some 180 physiotherapists in England and 141 in Australia completed the questionnaire. The questionnaire was designed to elicit: (a) background characteristics of participating physiotherapists, and (b) their reasons for choice of physiotherapy techniques.

The study involved the administration of a postal questionnaire to physiotherapists working in several hospitals in England and a comparison with several hospitals in Australia. The major difference between the two countries is that degree-level physiotherapy education has been instituted over the past two decades in Australia but it has commenced only recently in England.

A convenient sample was used, of hospital Trusts known to be centres for clinical education for physiotherapy in both the north and south of England, and in the Australian states of Victoria and Tasmania. The covering letters and questionnaires to individual respondents were distributed through physiotherapy department managers.

In England eight of the ten hospitals (80%) agreed to participate in the study, with 320 questionnaires being distributed and 180 completed, giving a response rate of 56%. In Australia 17 hospitals (81%) agreed to participate, with 240 questionnaires distributed and 141 completed and returned (59% response rate).

In the study, a major concern from the data was that, in both England and Australia, physiotherapists working in hospitals that provided training to student physiotherapists, and the qualified physiotherapists who conducted the questionnaire, indicated an extremely limited use of research or other journal literature as a basis for choice of treatment techniques. The benefit of degree-based education by experienced Australian physiotherapists seemed to have had little impact on promoting evidence-based practice; indeed, a startling feature of the study was the similarity of both national groups in their reasons for choosing techniques.

Source: Turner and Whitfield (1997).

Questions to ask of surveys

To help you appraise this form of evidence critically you may find the following questions helpful:

- How was the sample identified and selected?
- How was the questionnaire constructed; was an existing instrument used?

- What was the response rate?
- Was the issue of non-response bias addressed?
- Were all data reported?
- How was the questionnaire distributed?
- Were reminders included in the data collection process?

QUALITATIVE RESEARCH

The purpose of the range of qualitative methods is to understand phenomena in their natural environment. Qualitative research designs do not attempt to manipulate variables within the research setting (Patton, 1987) but are 'discovery oriented' (Guba and Lincoln, 1981). The process of enquiry attempts to understand naturally unfolding events within their context. Such a perspective is also finding growing expression as a range of healthcare professionals question the adequacy of attempting to explain how the world works by viewing it from a rationalistic perspective (Goodwin and Goodwin, 1984; Inui, 1996; Mishel, 1987).

The Evidence Example in Box 2.7 is of a study of the perceptions of recipients of a bone marrow transplant; it attempts to identify from their perspective the experience of transplantation. The data were collected through the process of in-depth interviews, which were audiotaped and transcribed verbatim. From these data the researchers undertook a process of content analysis from which five broad categories were identified.

While the construction of categories is an inherently subjective process, it remains perfectly possible for the researcher to make clear the rigour of the processes by which they emerge. The validity of qualitative methods is influenced by the skill, competence and rigour of the person undertaking the observation, as the observer is in effect the research instrument (Guba and Lincoln, 1981; Patton, 1987).

Reflection　From your own clinical experience take a moment to consider how you affect interview situations. Next time, try to reflect on how you act and react, the language you use and your verbal intonation. Then reflect on the Evidence Example in Box 2.7 and how the situation may have affected you.

The critical appraisal of qualitative research is about asking appropriate questions to interrogate the methodology as the means of analysis. While this process provides rich data in terms of informants' experiences, such as in the Evidence Example, the results have limited generalisability, representing as they do the experiences of only the individuals in the study. However, what does emerge from qualitative enquiry is the process of hypothesis generation. The researchers in the Evidence Example made clear that the categories that emerged could provide suggestions and direction for future research, which is an important part of the wider research picture.

Evidence Example: Qualitative Rearch

Box **2.7** Explanatory study of recipients' perceptions of bone marrow transplantation

Bone marrow transplantation (BMT) is now an established form of treatment for a wide range of malignant and non-malignant diseases. Research has led to understanding and effective treatment of many side-effects of BMT. However, relatively little is known about how patients perceive BMT, and how they view their experiences during transplantation.

The purpose of this study was to describe the perceptions of a small group of BMT recipients. Audiotaped interviews were undertaken with six recipients of BMT who were well and in remission. A convenient sample of informants was identified, which represented approximately 30% of the annual BMT workload in the study sites. Of the ten respondents, six were interviewed individually; of the potential respondents identified, two died, one relapsed and one did not respond. All consented to audiotape recording. None of the informants was known to the transcriber. Interviews lasted from 45 min to 1 h.

Interview tapes were transcribed verbatim and a latent content analysis applied, which allows the recognition and description of categories in the informant's conversation, resulting in 'thick description' of the data. Data were assigned to broad categories; the choice of naming categories was recognised as subjective.

This provided in-depth descriptive data of these individuals' experiences, which were analysed using latent content analysis. Five broad categories were identified under which data were grouped and discussed: mortality and death; luck; 'prison' (protective isolation); relationships; and physical effects. These revealed that patients attached relatively little importance to the physical effects of BMT, possibly because of the effectiveness of treatment.

However, this led to a focus on other concerns, which the categories reflect. The importance of family members, particularly spouses, in sharing the burden of BMT, and the strengthening of family relationships, were highlighted. The value of nurses was also emphasised. Protective isolation was found to be a stressor in two different ways. All of those interviewed reported concern with thoughts of their own mortality and possible death before and

Box 2.7 Cont'd

during BMT. Recommendations for nurses working in BMT units and suggestions for the direction of future research are made.

Source: Thain and Gibbons (1996).

Questions to ask of qualitative data

From clarifying the purpose of qualitative approaches to research it becomes possible to think through the most appropriate questions that should be asked of it. Try the following; you may want to add to them:

- Was the qualitative method that was used made clear in the aim of the study?
- Were the criteria for sample selection described clearly?
- What was the method of recruitment of participants?
- Was the sample random, purposeful, theoretical, convenient, census, quota or not stated?
- Does the paper describe the sample characteristics in terms of gender, ethnicity, social class, etc?
- Was the sample appropriate?
- Were the processes of fieldwork and the means of data collection described adequately?
- Was there a systematic approach to collecting data?
- How were the data subsequently analysed and interpreted?
- What evidence is there of attempts to establish validity and reliability of the findings?
- Do the findings reflect the phenomena accurately?
- Are they consistent over time and between researchers?

PROFESSIONAL CONSENSUS (GUIDELINES FROM ROYAL COLLEGES AND EXPERT GROUPS)

In many ways the concept of evidence-based practice presents an inherently appealing logic. Yet whilst the generation of knowledge adds to our understanding, it paradoxically increases our uncertainty and adds to the complexity of clinical decision making.

The knowledge base of an individual clinician is non-generalisable and rates very low within the CRD's hierarchy of evidence (see Box 2.2). The limitations of individuals to learn and retain all the knowledge necessary to inform professional practice becomes more acute as the volume of evidence expands (Weed, 1997). Part of the uncertainty in decision making is the cost of information processing. In his concept of bounded rationality Simon (1979) has shown that assumptions about rationality in decision making are unreasonable, that individuals value their information-processing costs more highly than we realise, often settling for a process of 'satisfying' in which they assess that their decision is good enough. Clinicians build experience in clinical judgement by drawing upon a range of sources to which they are selectively exposed.

Clinical experience and clinical expertise in practice may not relate to a whole population perspective, but only to that of the patients a clinician has seen. Specialisation can also result in a narrowing field of knowledge, which may bias the professional's judgement, adding to our 'misplaced faith in the unaided human mind' (Weed, 1997). The major pitfall of consensus is that it is often the loudest voice and most dominant personalities that prevail. The dynamics and structures of professional groups and differing traditions of enquiry also impose influences upon decisions. Whilst professional consensus and expert opinion has its place in providing valuable hunches and directions for much of research, it remains professional opinion. Not all decisions are capable of being based fully on research evidence; non-scientific mechanisms may more often influence clinical decision making than we acknowledge (McDonald, 1996). For this reason 'expert' review using independent researchers also has its limitations, for even experts come with their individual bias and values.

Reflection   Consider how you would define an 'expert'.

Questions to ask of professional consensus

As you can imagine, this is a difficult form of evidence to help you in critical appraisal. You should consider amongst other questions:

- How was 'expert' defined and by whom?
- What processes were used for the final decision-making agreement?
- Were any processes of external review undertaken?
- Who funded the process?

Clinical guidelines

As the use of clinical guidelines increases, so there is a need to be able to make judgements about their quality. The Health Care Evaluation Unit at St George's Hospital Medical School, London, undertakes the critical appraisal of guidelines on behalf of NHS Executive. A systematic approach is adopted using a critical appraisal instrument developed specifically for clinical guidelines. Increasingly this instrument is being adopted across Europe; it is freely available online at http://www.sghms.ac.uk/phs/hceu.

A FRAMEWORK OF QUESTIONS TO BE ASKED OF RESEARCH EVIDENCE

As you read around the subject of appraisal you will fine numerous frameworks of questions offered by authors. The example given here (Table 2.1) is from Benton and Cormack (1996).

Table 2.1 Questions to be asked of various sections of a research report	
Heading	**Question to be asked**
Title	Is the title concise? Is the title informative? Does the title clearly indicate the content? Does the title clearly indicate the research approach used?
Author(s)	Does the author(s) have appropriate academic qualifications? Does the author(s) have appropriate professional qualifications and experience?
Abstract	Is there an abstract included? Does the abstract identify the research problem? Does the abstract state the hypotheses (if appropriate)? Does the abstract outline the methodology? Does the abstract give details of the sample subjects? Does the abstract report major findings?
Introduction	Is the problem clearly identified? Is a rationale for the study stated? Are limitations of the study clearly stated?
Literature review	Is the literature up-to-date? Does the literature review identify the underlying theoretical framework(s)? Does the literature review present a balanced evaluation of material both supporting and challenging the position being proposed? Does the literature clearly identify the need for the research proposed? Are important references omitted?
The hypothesis	Does the study use an experimental approach? Is the hypothesis capable of testing? Is the hypothesis unambiguous?
Operational definitions	Are all terms used in the research question/problem clearly defined?
Methodology	Does the methodology section clearly state the research approach used? Is the method appropriate to the research problem?

Table 2.1 Cont'd	
Heading	**Question to be asked**
	Are the strengths and weaknesses of the chosen approach stated?
Subjects	Are the subjects clearly identified?
Sample selection	Is the sample selection approach congruent with the method to be used? Is the approach to sample selection clearly stated? Is the sample size clearly stated?
Data collection	Are any data collection procedures adequately described? Have the validity and reliability of any instruments or questionnaires been clearly stated?
Ethical considerations	If the study involves human subjects has the study received ethics committee approval? Is informed consent sought? Is confidentiality assured? Is anonymity guaranteed?
Results	Are results clearly presented? Are results internally consistent? Is sufficient detail given to enable the reader to judge how much confidence can be placed in the findings?
Data analysis	Is the approach appropriate to the type of data collected? Is any statistical analysis correctly performed? Is there sufficient analysis to determine whether 'significant differences' are not attributable to variation in other relevant variables? Is complete information (test value, degrees of freedom and probability) reported?
Discussion	Is the discussion balanced? Does the discussion draw upon previous research? Are the weaknesses of the study acknowledged? Are clinical implications discussed?
Conclusion	Are conclusions supported by the results obtained? Are the implications of the study identified?
Recommendations	Do the recommendations suggest further areas for research? Do the recommendations identify how any weaknesses in the study design could be avoided in future research?

From Benton and Cormack (1996), with permission.

EVIDENCE AND DECISION MAKING

Clinical decision making is a complex process, informed and influenced by a whole variety of factors, many of which are certainly not based on empirical evidence. As Klein (1996) has commented, scientific knowledge is only part of the complex process of clinical decision making, but dangers may be associated with the emphasis being placed upon 'new scientism' so that the most enthusiastic advocates of evidence-based healthcare may have failed to pay sufficient attention to the inherent uncertainty bound up in the process of clinical decision making. Not all of human life can be reduced to a unit of data in a RCT: indeed, the bias in the positivist paradigm itself reproduces a narrow scientism.

But evidence itself constantly evolves. Knowledge is always going to be incomplete and care will be delivered by inherently irrational, emotional, human beings, who on occasions make decisions for the most odd reasons. It is very difficult to disentangle the values attached to the processes of generating evidence, to take account of the values and tradition among different professional groups about the types of evidence. Studies of clinical behaviour often illustrate that there is a range of reasons behind a clinician's clinical judgement, as Turner and Whitfield (1997) have shown with physiotherapists. This is not unrelated to patient behaviour, as Petrie *et al.* (1996) have illustrated.

If this is the case, we need to know how to deal with situations in which best evidence is not always available, and in the numerous areas where there is a lack of 'strong' evidence. In the face of this situation the NHS Research and Development Programme has made a considerable investment in creating sources of synthesised evidence.

- The Cochrane library and Collaboration (web site and online access: http://www.cochrane.co.uk)
- NHS Centre for Reviews and Dissemination, University of York (see Chapter 3).

For all these resources access to libraries remains a problem for many healthcare staff; at the same time libraries are being called on to provide and present evidence in a range of forms, for a range of audiences (Roddham, 1995). In the White Paper *The New NHS: Modern, Dependable* (Department of Health, 1997), the Government has signalled clearly its commitment to the development of an NHS built on knowledge and the need to make high-quality knowledge widely available to more than just professional audiences.

GENERALISABILITY

To be able to apply evidence to similar practice settings from the original research setting makes an assumption about its generalisability. Can the results of a specific study be applied to the group of patients to whom you are applying these findings? In RCTs there are inevitably very tight inclusion and exclusion criteria for subjects in the study, for example no pre-existing disease or conditions. These criteria will, technically, limit the generalisability of the results, which would be applicable only to a similar group of patients. If the findings are applied to a wider group of patients, they are being generalised beyond the power of the study and used inappropriately. Hence, RCTs have also been described as representing the smallest unit of knowledge. Generalisability is the extent to which the findings of a study are applicable to the same phenomena in the wider population (LoBiondo-Wood, 1990), for example the use of low-dose aspirin in the treatment of myocardial infarction.

The authors of a study should make clear its limitations, yet this does not preclude readers of the work from applying it to other areas, and therefore the temptation is to overgeneralise findings.

The key issues across various types of evidence concern appropriate methods for the appropriate questions (da Vaus, 1993) and the rigour of the production process: transparency of the production method, inclusions, exclusions, claims of generalisability, not overstated, appropriately powered statistical analysis. Acknowledgement of limitations is highly appropriate: it is fine to have them, but they must be acknowledged.

BECOMING A DISCERNING CONSUMER

Reflection   The aim of this chapter has been to explore the different types of evidence that are available to you and how you can make judgements about their quality and usefulness. Take some time to reflect on the list of questions you made initially. Has your view of the quality of evidence changed in any way? As a consumer of research evidence, what might be the consequences of becoming more discerning?

As stated above, many research textbooks include a list of questions to ask of particular forms of evidence. The process of subjecting a piece of research to such questioning is known as critical appraisal. The key objective is to question critically the evidence that is being presented in order to make an informed judgement about its robustness and utility to your practice (LoBiondo-Wood, 1990).

Confidence in the use of evidence stems from you being able to judge the rigour of its production and applicability to your practice. The publication of research evidence in a reputable professional journal is not always a guarantee of its rigour. In recent years a number of cases of academic fraud, which is considered serious professional misconduct, have resulted in doctors being struck off of the medical register (Dyer, 1997). The editors of journals have also started to reflect on the processes by which they judge papers for publication (Smith, 1997). The process of peer review by professional journals is itself acknowledged as biased with questions of method and name bias, publication bias and values on differing traditions of enquiry (Wilkie, 1997). The relative usefulness and constraints of qualitative and quantitative evidence depend on the question you are asking; what is necessary is the appropriate method, and rigour in all matters.

Yet, despite all our attempts to find apparently rational solutions to the problems faced in clinical practice, we often fail to engage with the reality of practice. In a study of doctors in the USA, Canada and the UK, Greer (1988, p. 23), whose comments could equally have been made about a range of healthcare professionals, concluded that no matter how esteemed the research generators may be:

there are no magic signatories or formats which will cause knowledge to jump off the page and into practice. To incorporate new knowledge into their practices, physicians (sic) must feel comfortable with it, comfortable that it is true, applicable and supportable in the local community.

REFERENCES

Bale, S., Squires, D., Varnon, T., Walker A., Benbow, M. & Harding, K.G. (1997). A comparison of two dressings in pressure sore management. *Journal of Wound Care,* **6**(10), 463–466.

Benton, D. & Cormack, D. (1996). Reviewing and evaluating the literature. In *The Research Process in Nursing,* 3rd edn, ed. Cormack, D.F.S. pp. 78–87. Oxford: Blackwell Scientific.

Bircumshaw, D. (1990). The utilisation of research findings in clinical practice. *Journal of Advanced Nursing,* **15**, 1272–1280.

Brett, J.L. (1987). Use of nursing practice research findings. *Nursing Research,* **36**(6), 344–349.

Brookes, M. (1997). Lets hear it for failure. *New Scientist,* 15 March, 46.

Carter, D.E. (1996). Descriptive research. In *The Research Process in Nursing,* 3rd edn, ed. Cormack, D.F.S. pp. 179–189. Oxford: Blackwell Scientific.

Da Vaus, D.A. (1993). *Surveys in Social Research,* 3rd edn. London: UCL

Department of Health (1997). *The New NHS: Modern, Dependable.* London: The Stationery Office.

Dyer, C. (1997). Consultant struck off over research fraud. *British Medical Journal,* **315**, 205.

Eddy, D. (1988). The quality of medical evidence. *Health Affairs,* **Spring**, 20–32.

Freemantle, N. & Watt, I. (1994). Dissemination: implementing the findings of research. *Health Libraries Review,* **11**, 133–137

Goodwin, L.D. & Goodwin, W.L. (1984). Qualitative vs quantitative research or qualitative and quantitative research? *Nursing Research,* **33** (6), 378–380.

Greer, A.L. (1988). The state of the art versus the state of the science. *International Journal of Technology Assessment in Health Care,* **4**, 5–26.

Guba, E.G. & Lincoln, Y.S. (1981). *Effective Evaluation: Improving the Usefulness of Evaluation Through Responsive and Naturalistic Approaches.* New York: Josey Bass.

Haynes, R.B., Hayward, R.S.A. & Lomas, J. (1995). Bridges between health care research evidence and clinical practice. *Journal of the American Medical Information Association,* **2**, 342–350.

Inui, T.S. (1996). The virtue of qualitative and quantitive research. *Annals of Internal Medicine,* **125**(9), 770–771.

Kanouse, D.E. & Jacoby, I. (1988). When does information change practitioners' behaviour? *International Journal of Technology Assessment in Health Care,* **4**, 27–33.

Kendall, S. (1997). What do we mean by evidence? Implications for primary health care nursing. *Journal of Interprofessional Care,* **11**, 23–34.

Klein, R. (1996). The NHS and the new scientism: solution or delusion? *Quarterly Journal of Medicine,* **89**, 85–87.

LoBiondo-Wood, G.H.J. (1990). *Nursing Research: Methods, Critical Appraisal and Utilisation,* 2nd edn. St Louis: C.V. Mosby.

McDonald, C.J. (1996). Medical heuristics: the silent adjudicators of clinical practice. *Annals of Internal Medicine,* **124,** 56–62.

MacGuire, J. (1990). Putting nursing research into practice. *Journal of Advanced Nursing,* **15,** 614–620.

Macleod Clark, J. & Hockey, L. (1989). *Further Research for Nursing.* London: Scutari Press.

Milne, R. (1997). *Critical Appraisal Skills Programme.* Oxford: Centre for Evidence-based Medicine.

Mishel, M.H. (1987). Consider an alternative. *Heart and Lung,* **16**(3), 321–322.

Muir Gray, J.A. (1997). *Evidence-based Healthcare: How to Make Health Policy and Management Decisions.* London: Churchill Livingstone.

Norton, D. (1988). *Remembered with Advantage: Research Efforts Gone Before.* London: RCN.

Patton, M.Q. (1987). *How to Use Qualitative Methods in Evaluation.* Newbury Park, California: SAGE Publications.

Petrie, K.J., Weinman, J., Sharpe, N. & Buckley, J. (1996). Role of patients' view of their illness in predicting return to work and functioning after myocardial infarction: longitudinal study. *British Medical Journal,* **312,** 1191–1194.

Pocock, S.J. (1983). Publication and interpretation of findings. In: *Clinical Trials: A Practical Approach,* ed. Pocock, S.J. pp. 234–249. Chichester: J. Wiley.

Roberts, J., While, A. & Fitzpartick, J. (1995). Information-seeking strategies and data utilisation: theory and practice. *International Journal of Nursing Studies,* **32**(6), 601–611.

Roddham, M. (1995). Responding to the reforms –are we meeting the need? *Health Libraries Review,* **12,** 101–114.

St Leger, A.S.S.H.W.-B.J.P. (1992). *Evaluating Health Services' Effectiveness.* Milton Keynes: Open University Press.

Sheldon, T. & Chalmers, I. (1994). The UK Cochrane Centre and the NHS Centre for Reviews and Dissemination: respective roles within the Information Systems Strategy of the NHS R&D Programme, coordination and principles underlying collaboration. *Health Economics,* **3,** 201–203.

Simon, H. (1979). A behavioural model of rational choice. In: *Models of Thought,* ed. Simon, H., pp. 7–19. New Haven: Yale University Press.

Smith, R. (1997). Misconduct in research: editors respond. *British Medical Journal,* **315,** 201–202.

Taylor, G.D., Kirkland, T.A., McKenzie, M.M., Sutherland, B. & Wiens, R.M. (1995). The effect of surgical wound infection on postoperative hospital stay. *Canadian Journal of Surgery,* **38,** 149–153.

Thain, C.W. & Gibbons, B. (1996). An explanatory study of recipients' perceptions of bone marrow transplantation. *Journal of Advanced Nursing,* **23,** 528–535.

Turner, P. & Allan Whitfield, T.W. (1997). Physiotherapists' use of evidence based practice: a cross-national study. *Physiotherapy Research International,* **2,** 17–29.

Weed, L. (1997). New connections between medical knowledge and patient care. *British Medical Journal,* **315,** 231–235.

Wilkie, T. (1997). Sources in science: who can we trust? *Lancet,* **347,** 1308–1311.

Williamson, J.W., German, P.S., Weiss, R., Skinner, E.A. & Bowes, F. (1989). Health science information management and continuing education of physicians. *Annals of Internal Medicine,* **110**(2), 151–160.

3

Systematic reviews

Rumona Dickson

KEY ISSUES

◆ Systematic reviews provide the best evidence of effectiveness

◆ Good-quality systematic reviews are the result of a rigorous research process

◆ To make the best use of the evidence provided by a systematic review, healthcare providers need to be able to assess the quality of the review

◆ Systematic reviews do not provide all the information required to make clinical decisions but are an excellent point to begin your search for evidence

INTRODUCTION

Successful outcomes from the implementation of evidence-based practice depend on a combination of factors and activities. However, first and foremost, you need to know what works. The most effective implementation strategy will not produce positive results if it includes delivering an ineffective intervention. In the words of Muir Gray (1997, p. 17): 'We need to do the right things right'.

But perhaps we are a bit ahead of ourselves. Let us take time to examine some terms. If we accept the definition of evidence-based practice as the use of the best available evidence combined with clinical judgement (Sackett *et al.*, 1996; DiCenso, 1998), then we need to consider what constitutes best evidence. There are a number of methods that you can use to assess the evidence (Cook *et al.*, 1992). Historically, the most accessible to healthcare professionals has been research textbooks. Before the 1990s, the hierarchy of what was deemed 'best evidence' was headed by the results of randomised controlled trials. At its base may have been what key opinion leaders espoused. More recently, good quality systematic reviews have risen to the top of the list.

This chapter is designed to provide you with information about systematic reviews, what they are (and are not), their key components and how to assess their quality. The first part of the chapter describes what systematic reviews are. The second deals, in detail, with the components and process of conducting reviews. For some of you this will include more detail than you think you need (or perhaps want) but I believe it provides the necessary background for the final part of the chapter: assessing the quality of systematic reviews that contain information important to your clinical practice.

WHAT ARE SYSTEMATIC REVIEWS?

To begin this discussion it might be best to describe what systematic reviews are not. They are not what have traditionally been presented as literature reviews. We have all read these reviews and some of us have been part of the painful process of writing them. Historically, literature reviews were a vital part of the background to a research protocol, or a report of research results, or an academic paper. They often took a great deal of time to compile, but they varied in quality and in their ability to present an unbiased point of view. In fact, many made no attempt to be unbiased. In the time before computers and electronic databases, such reviews were begun by sifting a researcher's file-drawers and handsearching journals. An extensive search often meant consulting the files and memories of colleagues.

Times have changed. Systematic reviews are considered the 'gold standard' for assessing the effectiveness of a treatment or intervention (NHS Centre for Reviews and Dissemination, p. i 1996):

> Systematic reviews locate, appraise and synthesise evidence from scientific studies in order to provide informative, empirical answers to scientific research questions.

Put simply, this means that a systematic review brings together and assesses all available research evidence. This information can then be combined with your clinical judgement to make decisions about how to deliver the best care to your patients.

But is all this really necessary? Why have people spent so much time developing the process for conducting systematic reviews? The answer is quite simple. Given the amount and complexity of available information and the limitations of a health worker's time, there was a need to develop a process to provide, in a concise way, the results of research findings (Mulrow, 1995).

The vast amount of available research is discussed in other sections of this book. At the risk of repetition it is worth saying that the dramatic increase in the amount of available research makes it impossible for healthcare professionals to keep up to date – assuming, of course, that they have access to the information. A recent initiative by the Royal College of Nursing indicates that access, at least to some forms of information, is steadily decreasing in the UK (Casey, 1997).

Even if you do have access to the research literature, you have two further hurdles to cross. You need to be able to assess the quality of research reports. There are a number of resources available to help you develop the critical appraisal skills that you need to do this (Sackett *et al.*, 1991; Crombie, 1996). However, these skills take time and practice to develop and currently only a limited number of education programmes for health professionals include the teaching of critical appraisal skills in their curricula. Therefore, only a small proportion of healthcare workers develop the skills to assess the existing research objectively.

The second hurdle relates to the amount of available information. Even for a specific clinical problem, a large number of relevant studies may be found and the often conflicting report results need to be combined. Supposing you have the luxury of unlimited time, this process can still be daunting. Hence, the process of conducting systematic reviews has evolved and there has been an increase in the number of people conducting this type of research.

I would like to emphasise that I am referring here to systematic reviews that are designed to assess effectiveness. Does a treatment or intervention work? Does it do more good than harm? With this in mind we need to be sure that the studies included in such reviews provide us with the least biased results. Historically this has meant reviews that include only randomised controlled trials, that is studies that ensure it was the intervention that had an effect on the outcome and not some other extraneous factor(s). There has been a lot of debate about the value of using the results of studies other than randomised controlled trials (Sackett and Wennberg, 1998). I do not intend to contribute to that debate here except to say two things. The first is that we cannot ignore the value of reviews that use less rigorous evidence. However, the value of such reviews is not in providing evidence of effectiveness but in clarifying current levels of knowledge and in directing the design of future research.

With this as background, let us now move on to more specific information about the process of doing a systematic review.

HOW ARE SYSTEMATIC REVIEWS CONDUCTED?

Just for an instant – well, maybe more than an instant – let us say that you are thinking about conducting a systematic review to assess the effectiveness of a current treatment practice. How would you go about it? Where would you start?

It is clear, given the definition of a systematic review, that conducting a review is a research process and that it requires adherence to a strict scientific protocol (NHS Centre for Reviews and Dissemination, 1996). Therefore, in the same way as you would begin any research project by defining your research question and your methodology in a research protocol, you must do the same for a systematic review The components that should be addressed in the protocol are included in Box 3.1.

I know that most of you will never carry out a systematic review. But you do need to know how to assess the quality of a systematic review to inform your practice. To be able to carry out this quality assessment you require an understanding of how a high-quality review is conducted. So we will continue to imagine that you are going to do a systematic review and examine the activities that go with each of the components listed in Box 3.1.

Definition of the research question

Defining the question is the most important activity in conducting a systematic review. Failure to take the time to formulate a clearly defined question at the beginning of the review means wasting a great deal of your own time and that of anyone who tries to use the review. The question provides the direction for the carrying out of the other activities of the review (Mulrow and Oxman, 1994). Your question should include a definition of the participants, the intervention(s) to be assessed and the outcomes to be measured.

Vague questions lead to vague and often poor-quality reviews. For example, the question 'What can we do to decrease injuries to the elderly?' is very broad and does not clearly specify exactly what it is you want to examine. A more specifically focused question such as 'Do exercise

Box **3.1** Key components of the systematic review process

1. Definition of the research question
2. Methods for identifying research studies
3. Selection of studies for inclusion
4. Quality appraisal of included studies
5. Extraction of the data
6. Synthesis of the data

interventions prevent falls among the elderly?' provides us with an intervention (exercise), a participant group (the elderly) and an outcome (falls).

If you begin to read a systematic review and it is not based on a clearly defined question, you are unlikely to get a clear answer. You may, therefore, wish to spend your valuable time in a more productive way. We will discuss this later in the context of quality assessment of systematic reviews.

Once you are satisfied with the question then you can proceed to lay out your plan of action.

Methods for identifying research studies

Although a brief literature search and knowledge of the subject area are needed to define the research question, the actual review is based on a comprehensive search of the literature. You will need to identify both published and unpublished material (theses, conference proceedings, special reports) as well as material in languages other than English. The purpose of such a broad search is to limit, as much as possible, the bias of the review.

So where will you begin? Box 3.2 contains the elements of a comprehensive search strategy.

Database searching

Database are a valuable tool in the search process. They allow access to large amounts of literature, provide an estimate of how much information is available and often provide information, in abstract form, that can help reviewers to make a preliminary assessment of studies. However, more than 200 databases exist and searching them is not to be taken lightly.

When selecting the specific database(s) to search, you will need to consider which journals are listed on the database, how the publications are

---

Box 3.2 Elements of the search strategy

- Database searching
- Handsearching
- Searching reference lists of identified studies
- Contacting researchers in the field
- Finding unpublished literature

indexed, your access to the database and any cost implications. It is unlikely that one database will list all the journals you want to search. Therefore, you will likely need to search more than one database. Databases differ not only in the journals they index, but in how the indexing is done. This means that you need to design a new search strategy for each database.

Database searching should be considered as only one component of the literature search and its limitations need to be recognised (Dickson and Sindhu, 1997). A specific example of these limitations has been provided by Dickersin and Min (1993). They compared the results of handsearching with electronic searching of MEDLINE. Their electronic search of selected journals failed to identify 12% of the trials that had been found through handsearching of the same journals.

Handsearching

Handsearching identifies studies in journals that may not have been indexed on an electronic database, or may have been indexed in such a way that database searching is impractical. Comprehensive handsearching requires knowledge of the subject area and of the journals most likely to publish the research you are trying to find. There are two decisions to be made before you begin: (1) which journals should you search and (2) how far back do you search?

Which journals you handsearch depends on the research question (remember, a good review is directed by a clear and concise research question). If the topic is narrow, then as few as four or five journals may meet your needs. However, if the topic is broad or is addressed by journals from several disciplines (e.g. nursing, medicine and/or physiotherapy) then the list of journals to be handsearched may be longer. In a review of the non-pharmacological management of pain, for example, the author hand-searched 52 journals (Sindhu, 1996). The aim is to use your time efficiently by identifying the journals you think will contain the most relevant studies.

How many years of each journal you search also depends on the research question. For instance, if you are conducting a review of a relatively new treatment, you may need to search only the past few years. However, if you are comparing the effectiveness of an intervention that has been in use for a long time, you may need to search across a wider range of years.

For those with an interest in the details of handsearching (I realise the numbers will be limited), the most extensive strategy I have come across is included in a recent book (Graham, 1997). The book is a history of the use of episiotomy (it is not specifically a review of effectiveness). The search includes 10 journals and extends back to 1868. But take heart, this is the exception and not the rule.

Once you have identified the journals you believe need to be hand-searched, you need to locate them physically. This is not always as easy as it sounds. It is an unwritten rule of systematic reviews that, if you need to find two journals, they are likely to be in two different libraries many miles apart. Having located the journals, you simply check each volume to see whether it contains studies that seem to meet the inclusion criteria of your review. You then photocopy these studies and they go into the selection process for studies set out in the protocol of your review (see Selection of studies for inclusion below).

Checking reference lists

No matter how studies are identified for inclusion in the review, you will need to check the bibliography of each one to identify other studies that might meet your review inclusion criteria. This can be a very valuable exercise. In a recent review on the treatment of intestinal parasites (worms) in children five of the 27 included studies were identified by checking the reference list of other studies included in the review (Dickson *et al.*, 1999).

Contacting researchers in the field

One of the best, and at times most enjoyable, ways of identifying ongoing or unpublished studies is to contact researchers in the field of interest. However, the process is time consuming and can be costly. There is no best way to carry out this part of the literature search (McGrath, Davies and Soares, 1998). You may choose to contact researchers by telephone, post or e-mail. The attitude of researchers to systematic reviews varies and, since you may be asking them to spend their valuable time in assisting you with your review, they may not always welcome you with open arms (Roberts and Schierhout, 1997). On the other hand, many researchers are happy to share their information and can add valuable information to your review. You may also be fortunate enough to come in contact with other researchers conducting similar work, and other collaborative projects may result from your efforts. Another positive outcome of this personal contact may be that you identify researchers who are willing to provide feedback for you on draft and final copies of your review.

Finding unpublished literature

There is no standard method for identifying unpublished studies. They may be included in Masters' or PhD theses which may or may not be listed on a database. They may feature in conference proceedings. Just as you spent time identifying which journals to handsearch, you may need to spend time identifying the conferences at which relevant papers may have been presented. You may be able to obtain these from professional organisations or through your contacts with researchers in the field. The identification of unpublished studies is critical because it is the best way of decreasing bias, which may be introduced if you include only published material.

Bias

As stated above, the reason for conducting a comprehensive search of the literature is to identify as much of the available information as possible. Failure to do so can potentially bias the results of the review. Since decreasing the effects of bias in reviews is important, this seems a good time to discuss a few forms of bias which could be introduced through your search.

With the explosion of work in systematic reviews, interest has arisen in components of the reviews that may be biased by the review activities themselves. Since review results are based on studies you identify with your search strategy, you need to be aware of how bias might affect what you find. Egger and Davey Smith (1998) have described a number of these factors in detail. Here I will touch on only a few.

We know that a great deal of completed research is never reported in research journals (Easterbrook *et al.*, 1991, Dickersin and Min, 1993). This is particularly true in nursing and the reasons are multifaceted (Hicks, 1995). Writing up research findings is challenging and time consuming, so researchers are less motivated to write up the results of studies that do not produce significant findings. Editors of research journals are also less likely to publish the results of studies with non-significant findings. This means that published studies are more likely to report significant positive or negative findings. Obviously, if you include only published work in the review, this bias can have a potentially dramatic effect on the results of the review.

A recent initiative has been launched to identify unpublished trials (Smith and Roberts, 1997). Encouraged by researchers conducting systematic reviews, this is being supported by more than 100 journals around the world. Researchers are being asked to submit details of their unpublished research, and this information will be made available on the Internet and thus be available for inclusion in systematic reviews.

It is easier for English-speaking researchers to identify and gain access to research results published in English. It is also true that researchers are more likely to publish significant positive findings in English language journals, thus creating a language bias (Moher *et al.*, 1996).

All of these factors could have an effect on the quality of your systematic review and should be considered when you are designing your search strategy.

Selection of studies for inclusion

The criteria used to select studies for inclusion in the review are critical to its outcome and they should be defined before you begin your literature search. This helps to ensure that your criteria are not based on the research results that you know are available.

The concept of inclusion criteria can be confusing and it may help if I use an analogy. If you were to carry out a trial on the effectiveness of a new drug for hypertension you would need to define what patients were to be included in your study. Therefore, before you see any patients you would set your criteria. These might state, for example, that participants will be male and female patients, aged between 45 and 65 years, with a diastolic pressure greater than 110mmHg. Each time you see a patient you will then assess them to see whether they meet the criteria and therefore will be invited to take part in the trial. This has nothing to do with which group they may be assigned to in the trial itself – it deals only with their eligibility to enter it.

In the same way as you would not gather a group of patients in a room and look them over to see which ones to include in your hypertension trial, you would not collect a pile of studies and, on seeing what they contain, decide whether you will include them in the review. This seems to be commonsensical but, since many reviewers are clinical experts familiar with research in the field, it can prove difficult to exclude personal biases when defining inclusion criteria.

The inclusion criteria that you set should be a direct reflection of the research question, which includes the participants, the intervention and the outcomes (Table 3.1). The one additional component of the inclusion criteria is the type of studies that will be included in the review and, since we are talking about reviews of effectiveness, these will be randomised or pseudorandomised controlled trials.

By explicitly defining the inclusion criteria for the review, the activity of study selection becomes very transparent; that is, anyone should be able to look at a study and see why it was, or was not, included in the review.

One other point is that your review protocol may also explicitly list exclusion criteria. This may help both the reviewers and the readers of the review. So, in the example in Table 3.1, a given exclusion criterion said that the review would exclude any studies that only reported effects on the number of parasites found in the children. This tells readers interested in the effectiveness of the drugs on specific parasites that they will not find such information in this review.

We know, of course, that individuals may interpret the same research report in slightly different ways. It is valuable, therefore, to have more than one reviewer independently apply the inclusion criteria to each study. These reviewers should then meet and compare their decisions and discuss

	Table 3.1 Selection criteria determined by the research question: What is the effect of anthelminthic drug treatment in children in relation to their growth or cognitive performance? (Translation: Do children grow and learn better if you rid them of intestinal worms?)		
	Research question	**Inclusion criteria**	**Exclusion criteria**
Participants	Children	Children aged 1–16 years	
Intervention	Drug treatment	Treatment with any drug currently listed in the *British National Formulary* for treatment of intestinal parasites delivered at any location (school, clinic, community)	
Outcomes	Nutritional status	Growth measures (height, weight, anthropometric measures)	Studies that measured only parasite rates (e.g. egg counts)
	Cognitive performance	Any test of cognition	
Type of study	Not listed in question	Any randomised or pseudorandomised controlled trial	

any discrepancies. A mediator is sometimes helpful to assist in the discussion of these discrepancies.

The defining and application of appropriate inclusion criteria are critical to the quality and value of a given review. Once you have applied them and the studies are selected, the next step is to assess the quality of the included studies.

Quality appraisal of included studies

The usefulness of any systematic review is largely dependent on the quality of studies included in it. Therefore, even if your inclusion criteria state that all studies will be randomised controlled trials, you must examine further each of these included trials to see whether they were high-quality studies. As we all know, not all research is conducted using the best possible methods or, in the words of a colleague, 'not all randomised controlled trials are created equal'.

Just as you would examine each patient in a trial to assess whether their current health status might affect their response to treatment, each study in your review must be assessed for the quality of its research methodology. Poorly conducted trials provide unreliable and often biased results.

There are numerous criteria and checklists designed to assess the quality of a randomised controlled trial (Moher *et al.*, 1995). It is not the purpose of this chapter to describe these in detail. However, it is important to understand the factors in the trial design that may bias the review.

A major form of bias that can be introduced into a randomised controlled trial may arise if the researchers are aware of the group to which individuals will be assigned if they come into the trial. This knowledge may bias them for or against recruiting a patient. For example, in a study of leg ulcer care, if the healthcare professional is aware of the sequence of allocation and that the person being recruited will be put in the placebo group, they may not recruit them. Bias could also be introduced if the researcher recruits the person because they know they will be allocated to the placebo group.

What does this mean to the results of trials? Schulz and colleagues (1995) studied 250 controlled trials and found that, if there was inadequate concealment of allocation (i.e. that recruiters might have been able to tell which group a patient would be assigned to on entering the trial), the treatment effects of the trial were shown to be greater. In the same investigation, trials with inadequate sequence generation (e.g. they used alternate assignment such as dates of birth or dates of admission instead of random number tables to allocate patients) also showed greater effects.

Another factor to be addressed concerns including all participants in analysis of trial results. At the end of the trial, data for all those randomised to participate should be included in results or an explanation provided for any patients who dropped out, could not be found or died. Excluding results from some trial participants can change the researchers' conclusions. For example, in our leg ulcer trial, what happens if 25% of those in the treatment arm of the trial drop out because they do not think it is helping and their data are not included in the results? Obviously, if the reported results include only those who were helped by the treatment and therefore continued the treatment, the study may have false-positive results.

These are only three quality factors that may affect the results of the primary research. So why are they important in a systematic review? Bias in the primary research creates bias in the systematic review and may influence its findings and recommendations. If none of the studies shows properly concealed allocation, you know that these studies will show greater effects and you have a biased results.

What you do with the information you gain from the quality assessment of included studies is another issue. There are a number of things you can do. You can ignore it. You can decide to exclude the poor-quality trials, or you can include all the studies, do your analysis and then redo the analysis with the poor-quality studies removed (sensitivity analysis). The decision is not an easy one and in part will depend on the number of trials in your review, their overall quality and your area of study. What is important is that you establish and make known to your readers the methods you used to assess the quality of the trials and how you then incorporated that information in the data analysis.

Extraction of the data

As you develop the protocol for your review you define the outcomes of importance to you and your clinical decisions. You then need to identify how you will get that information from the included studies. There are numerous possible methods. The important factor is that the data are extracted as accurately as possible and in a manner that makes them easy to use when you begin your analysis.

To do this you may choose to design a data-extraction form on which you will record the information from each trial included in the review. It is worthwhile pilot-testing a few different styles of the form to see which works best for recording the data and which is also easy to use when you are working with the data for your analysis. Accuracy is very important. Accepted practice is that at least two people be involved in the extraction of data from included studies. It may be that each reviewer extracts data from all the included trials and then the data are cross-checked, or each reviewer could extract data from a portion of the trials and cross-check the data extracted by the other reviewer.

Synthesis of the data

Now that you have a plan for getting the data, what will you do with it? As in other high-quality research it is important that you define the analysis in the review protocol, before collecting the data. This means that you will have initial hypotheses that you want to test. Just as it is inappropriate to collect data in a field trial and to see what comes up before deciding on the analysis to be carried out, it is also inappropriate in a systematic review. Even worse is to carry out all possible comparisons and then report only those with significant findings.

For example, in the review into the effect of parasite drug treatment on child growth, the growth measures were defined as height, weight and skinfold measures. The analyses outlined in the protocol included comparing the average and changes in these measures for treated and non-treated children.

Data from a review can be analysed in several ways. Sometimes it will be quantitative in nature and lend itself to a statistical test called 'meta-analysis'. This is a statistical method of combining data from independent studies (Egger and Davey, 1997; Egger, Davey Smith and Phillips, 1997). It is a complex task and a great deal of thought needs to go into the comparisons to be made, the type of data to be used and, most importantly, whether it makes sense to combine data from different studies (Lau, Ioannidis and Schmid, 1997). It is not the purpose of this chapter to provide the information you need to understand meta-analysis (nor am I the person to do so). The section on quality appraisal of systematic reviews presents some questions you should consider when looking at a meta-analysis. What is most important is to consider whether it is appropriate to combine the findings from different studies.

In any event, the findings of much of today's research do not lend themselves to statistical analysis. It may be that the data have not been reported in a way that allows for meta-analysis. For example, the researchers may have weighed the children and measured their height but report the results as an aggregate measure of weight-for-height. In this case you cannot calculate the average weight or height of children and are not able to include the data in the statistical analysis. Or it may be that the data are qualitative in nature. Therefore, some, or all, of a analysis may be presented in the form of a narrative summary of the findings. This is a difficult task and it can prove difficult to limit the bias that can be introduced. Just as you define beforehand the quantitative analysis to be carried out in the review, you need to consider some *a priori* comparisons for qualitative data. This usually includes discussions about appropriate data to be extracted and the way in which tables might be set up to present and compare the available information.

So, have I totally discouraged you from doing a systematic review? I hope not. But, let us be realistic. Most of you will have little interest in carrying out a systematic review. So why should you be bothered with them? Because you want to deliver the best care possible and to do this you need to know what are the most effective interventions. Such information is available in systematic reviews. So, even if you never do a systematic review, you need to know how to assess their quality so that you can decide on whether to believe their results and integrate the findings into your clinical practice. The last section of this chapter deals with issues around deciding whether a given review has been conducted in a manner likely to produce reliable findings. The implementation of those findings will be dealt with later in this book.

JUDGING THE QUALITY OF A SYSTEMATIC REVIEW

You have just had a meeting with your supervisor to discuss nursing strategies for addressing the issue of patient falls in your clinical area.

Later that day you receive a copy of a systematic review that addresses this issue (Joanna Briggs Institute for Evidence Based Nursing and Midwifery, 1998). Your supervisor wants to know, given the findings in the review, whether you should consider a change in your clinical practice. Where do you begin?

First, a word of caution: in my experience of introducing nurses, physiotherapists and occupational therapists to systematic reviews, they show a fairly consistent initial response. They first look at the abstract and then look at the tables before saying, 'There are too many statistics here and I don't understand statistics'. They assume that they will not be able to understand the review, although this is patently untrue. Having read the first part of this chapter you will have all the information you need to judge whether you have a high-quality review. If it is, then you can find someone to help you decide whether the statistical analysis is correct. Do not allow yourself to be boggled by the statistics.

Earlier in the chapter we discussed the key components of a systematic review. A number of authors have developed strategies for assessing the quality of a given systematic review (Oxman, 1994; Song, 1994; Mulrow, 1995). In this section we will use a combination of these examples (Box 3.3).

Does the review have a well-defined question?

You know that conducting a systematic review is a research process driven by a research question and that such questions need to address three key issues: (1) Who are the participants? (2) What is done to them? and (3) What outcomes are assessed? So, the first thing you need to do is to

---

Box 3.3 Assessing the quality of a systematic review

1. Does the review have a well-defined question?

2. Has a substantial effort been made to search the literature?

3. Are the inclusion and exclusion criteria described and do they seem appropriate?

4. Do the authors tell you whether they assessed the quality of the studies included in the review?

5. Do the authors give you sufficient information about individual studies?

6. Have they combined the studies appropriately?

examine the review to see whether the author(s) have indeed presented you with a well-defined question. If they have not, if you cannot really tell who the participants in the studies are or exactly what the interventions are or what outcomes were measured, then it is not likely that you will get a clear answer to your question. If you were reading this review for your enjoyment, you might well decide not to use your time reading the rest of it. However, in this situation you have to report back to your supervisor, so let us continue.

Has a substantial effort been made to search the literature?

We described in some detail how literature searches are carried out and the importance of such searches in decreasing the bias of the review. What you need to do is to examine the search strategy that the author(s) describe and judge whether you think it will identify all the relevant literature. Things to ask yourself are: (1) Have they searched appropriate databases? (2) Did they use appropriate keywords in the search strategy? and (3) Did they attempt to identify unpublished literature? Since this review is in your clinical area of expertise, you will have a good idea of the important studies in the area. If the reviewers failed to identify a study that you believe should have been included, then perhaps their search was not as comprehensive as it might have been.

Are the inclusion and exclusion criteria described and do they seem appropriate?

The first step in this part of the assessment is related to whether the reviewers tell you, in clear terms, what criteria they used to make decisions about which studies were included in the review. This description should include the participants, the interventions, the outcome measures and the type of studies. One way to judge whether this has been described adequately is to imagine that you have just received a copy of a new research report. Given the criteria provided within the review, would you be able to decide whether this new study should be included in the review?

The second step requires your clinical judgement. The reviewers may have described their criteria adequately, but do they make sense? Are they appropriate? The area that causes the most problems is the outcome measures. Historically, research has been designed to measure clinically important outcomes (a drop in blood pressure, a change in weight). These outcomes are not always the ones that are important to you or your patients. Of course, this may not be the fault of the review, but a limitation of the basic research that is has been carried out.

Do the authors tell you whether they assessed the quality of the studies included in the review?

The quality of the review can only be as good as the quality of the studies that are included in it. It is important to know whether and how the reviewers examined the quality of the trials within the review and how they used that information in the analysis. For example, if they had a large number of poor-quality trials, did they include them in the analysis?

Do the authors give you sufficient information about individual studies?

The minimum information that should be made available for each included study is the design, the sample size, a description of the intervention, and the outcomes. You need this information to decide whether the studies met the inclusion criteria and also to judge whether the participants in the included trials are similar to one another and to the patients you encounter in your clinical practice.

Have they combined the studies appropriately?

This is where you might need or want some help from a statistician. But before you call one you should examine the comparisons that the reviewers have made and see whether they make sense. Were the studies similar enough so that it makes sense to combine the results? If you have taken a basic course in statistics, you may also be able to make some preliminary judgements about the statistics and what they mean.

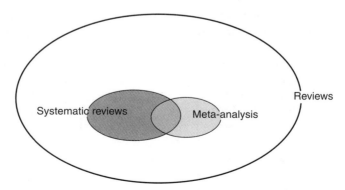

Figure 3.1 Relationship between traditional literature reviews, systematic reviews and meta-analysis.

There is one further point to be made about the use of meta-analysis. Just because a report uses meta-analysis to combine the data does not mean that the meta-analysis is based on a systematic review. This is important because the authors of such a paper may simply have combined the results of their favourite five or six studies. If they have a biased selection of studies in their analysis, they cannot help but come up with a biased result. Figure 3.1 shows the relationship between traditional literature reviews, systematic reviews and meta-analysis.

Having answered these six questions, you have systematically examined all the major components of the review. You can now make a judgement about whether you think it is a high-quality review and whether the findings are valid. The next decision is whether the findings should be incorporated into your clinical practice. This is not an easy task as there are numerous factors to be considered. Even when you have decided, based on the findings in a review, that you should implement changes to your practice, there may be influential external forces that will affect your ability to do so (Dickson *et al.*, 1998). But that is the topic for another chapter.

CONCLUSION

In this chapter I have discussed the major activities involved in conducting a systematic review. I have also supplied a set of questions to use in assessing the quality of such reviews. I hope this information will prove to be valuable as you encounter systematic reviews as a part of your clinical practice.

I would like to add one comment, and that is to say that systematic reviews will not answer all of your clinical questions. They are not guidelines to practice. Systematic reviews are designed to present the best available evidence in relation to a specific area of care or treatment. You and your colleagues need to take this evidence, incorporate it with your clinical judgement and information from individual patients, and make a plan that will deliver the best possible care.

This process can be broken down into a number of activities. These include identification of a clinical problem, identification and assessment of the available evidence, and decision making related to future clinical activities. As with introducing you to systematic reviews, I do not want to be discouraging but I will caution you that taking on the activities outlined in the box will require time and dedication. However, the process can be exciting and the rewards of carrying such a project to completion can be great for you, your colleagues and the people who depend on you for their care.

Table 3.2 Programme of activities for assessing clinical practice

Action steps	Notes
1. Identify a clinical problem in which you believe you may not be providing the best possible care. This identification should outline what care you currently provide.	Start small. Make the topic something that you, as a group, can likely do something about (e.g. decreasing patient falls, delivery of preoperative patient education, strategies for managing fever in children).
2. Carry out a literature search to see whether a systematic review has been carried out or any randomised controlled trials published. It is good if you have a group of people so you can divide up the work here. Use Appendix I to decide what data sources may be the best to meet your needs.	Preventing falls in hospital has been reviewed (Joanna Briggs Institute for Evidence Based Nursing and Midwifery, 1998). There is at least one good review in the area of preoperative teaching (Devine, 1992). A group in Perth is carrying out a review in the area of fever and children (protocol available on website: www.joannabriggs.edu.au/members/protofu.html).
3. Bring the results of the search to the group and discuss the quality of the research.	Each person should have read every article before you get together but it is often more productive if one person is responsible for leading the discussion. If your group needs some help in assessing the quality of the research you may want to invite an external expert to provide some guidance (e.g. clinical research nurse, research development officer, faculty member from a local university).
4. Compare the research findings to your clinical area and decide whether there are changes that you would like to implement in light of the evidence.	Now the challenging part really begins.

The steps in Table 3.2 are adapted from a successful programme that was carried out in two hospitals. Groups of nurses from six different clinical areas worked with a nursing research facilitator over the period of 1 year to get to step 4 (M. Edwards, personal communication).

REFERENCES

Casey, N. (1997). Library access: campaigning for better information (editorial). *Nursing Standard*, **12**(6), 1.

Cook, D., Guyatt, G., Laupacis, A. & Sackett, D. (1992). Rules of evidence and clinical recommendations on the use of antithrombotic agents. *Chest*, **102**, 305S–311S.

Crombie, I. (1996). *The Pocket Guide to Critical Appraisal*. London: BMJ Publishing Group.

Devine, E. (1992). Effects of psycho-educational care for adult surgical patients: a meta-analysis of 191 studies. *Patient Education and Counselling*, **19**, 129–142.

DiCenso, A. (1998). Implementing evidence-based nursing: some misconceptions. *Evidence-Based Nursing*, **1**(2), 38–40.

Dickersin, K. & Min, Y. (1993). NIH clinical trials and publication bias. *On-line Journal of Current Clinical Trials* (serial online), 28 April (50).

Dickson, R. & Sindhu, F. (1997). The complexity of searching the literature. *International Journal of Nursing Practice*, 3 (4), 211–218.

Dickson, R., Abdullahi, D., Flores, W. *et al.* (1998). Putting evidence into practice: developing approaches that use systematic reviews. *World Health Forum*, **19**, 311–314.

Dickson, R., Awasthi, S., Demmellweek, C. & Williamson, P. (1999). Anthelminthic therapy in children – effects on growth and cognitive performance. *The Cochrane Library*, Issue 1.

Easterbrook, P., Berlin, J., Gopalan, R. & Mathews, D. (1991). Publication bias in clinical research. *Lancet*, **337**, 867–872.

Egger, M. & Davey, S.G. (1997). Meta-analysis: potentials and promise. *British Medical Journal*, **315**, 1371–1374.

Egger, M. & Davey Smith, G. (1998). Bias in location and selection of studies. *British Medical Journal*, **316**, 61–66.

Egger, M., Davey Smith, G. & Phillips, A. (1997). Meta-analysis: principles and procedures. *British Medical Journal*, **315**, 1533–1537.

Graham, I. (1997). *Episiotomy: Challenging Obstetric Interventions*. Oxford: Blackwell.

Hicks, C. (1995). The shortfall in published research: a study of nurses' research publication activities. *Journal of Advanced Nursing*, **21**, 594–604.

Joanna Briggs Institute for Evidence Based Nursing and Midwifery (1998). *Falls in Hospital – Best Practice Information Sheet*. Adelaide: Joanna Briggs Institute for Evidence Based Nursing and Midwifery.

Lau, J., Ioannidis, J. & Schmid, C. (1997). Quantitative synthesis in systematic reviews. *Annals of Internal Medicine*, **127**(9), 820–826.

McGrath, J., Davies, G. & Soares, K. (1998). Writing to authors of systematic reviews elicited further data in 17% of cases. *British Medical Journal*, **316**, 631.

Moher, D., Jadad, A., Nichol, G., Penman, M., Tugwell, P. & Walsh, S. (1995). Assessing the quality of randomized controlled trials: an annotated bibliography of scales and checklists. *Controlled Clinical Trials*, **6**, 62–73.

Moher, D., Fortin, P., Jadad, A. *et al.* (1996). Completeness of reporting of trials published in languages other than English: implications for conduct and reporting of systematic reviews. *Lancet*, **347**, 363–366.

Muir Gray, J. (1997). *Evidence-based Health Care. How to Make Health Policy and Management Decisions*. London: Churchill Livingstone.

Mulrow, C. (1995). Rationale for systematic reviews. In *Systematic Reviews*, ed. Chalmers, I. & Altman, D. pp. 1–8. London: BMJ Publishing Group.

Mulrow, C. & Oxman, A.E. (1994). *The Cochrane Handbook*. Oxford: The Cochrane Collaboration.

NHS Centre for Reviews and Dissemination (1996). *Undertaking Systemic Reviews for Research Effectiveness: CRD Guidelines for Those Carrying Out and Commissioning Reviews*. University of York: NHS Centre for Reviews and Dissemination.

Oxman, A. (1994). Checklists for review articles. *British Medical Journal*, **309**, 648–651.

Roberts, I. & Schierhout, G. (1997). The private life of systematic reviews. *British Medical Journal*, **315**, 686–87.

Sackett, D. & Wennberg, J. (1998). Choosing the best research design for each question (editorial). *British Medical Journal,* **315**, 1636.

Sackett, D., Haynes, R., Guyatt, D. & Tugwell, P. (1991). *Clinical Epidemiology: A Basic Science for Clinical Medicine.* Toronto: Little, Brown.

Sackett, D., Rosenberg, W., Gray, J., Haynes, R. & Richardson, W. (1996). Evidence based medicine: what it is and what it isn't. *British Medical Journal,* **312**, 71–72.

Schulz, K., Chalmers, I., Hayes, R. & Altman, D. (1995). Dimensions of methodological quality associated with estimates of treatment effects in controlled trials. *Journal of the American Medical Association,* **273** (5), 408–412.

Sindhu, F. (1996). Are non-pharmacological nursing interventions for the management of pain effective: a meta-analysis. *Journal of Advanced Nursing* **24**, 1152–1159.

Smith, R. & Roberts, I. (1997). An amnesty for unpublished trials. *British Medical Journal,* **315**, 622.

Song, F. (1994). *Checklist for Quality Assessment of Published Reviews.* York: NHS Centre for Reviews and Dissemination, University of York.

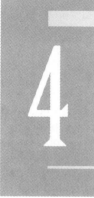

Information sourcing

Judith Palmer & Anne Brice

KEY ISSUES

◆ Factors that contribute to the 'information problem'

◆ Understanding the impact of information-seeking behaviour

◆ The range and relevance of sources of information

◆ How a structured approach to searching for evidence can provide
a sound basis for evidence-based practice and reduce the
'information problem' to manageable proportions

INTRODUCTION

Information is an intrinsic part of all decision making and problem solving. Healthcare problems may be addressed in many ways. There is seldom a single or an obvious direct route to a possible solution. The particular approach chosen will often depend as much on personality, previous experience and present resources as on information input (Martyn, 1987). For many healthcare professionals 'information' represents 'a problem'. To locate information it may be necessary to use many sources, animate and inanimate, and to evaluate these sources. Information may be scant or may be so abundant as to overwhelm; once found, it may be shared, hoarded, ignored or discarded. If retained, it must be stored in such a way as to be retrievable later. Some information declines in importance with age, other accrues lustre; some information is useful on its own, other only in coexistence or conjunction. Few people find information easily; many complain about the rigidity and rule-bound nature of information retrieval systems, both manual and electronic. Some struggle with catalogues, keywords and indexes, but for many it often seems easier to telephone a colleague or abandon the search.

THE INFORMATION PROBLEM

Quantity and quality

The exponential rise in the scientific literature is well documented. In a classic study in the early 1960s, Price (1963) showed that this trend has existed since the early eighteenth century and is not a modern phenomenon. In biomedicine it has been estimated that the literature doubles every 19 years (Wyatt, 1991). The past 5 years has seen a similar exponential rise in the number of World Wide Web sites on the Internet. It is estimated that in June 1993 there were 130 web sites, whereas in January 1997 this number had increased to 650,000 (Lynch, 1997). Information overload is a daily reality for all health professionals as they struggle to cope, not only with the published literature, but also with an avalanche of electronic mail, information from Internet bulletin boards, newsgroups, discussion lists and other electronic information sources. Apart from the quantity of published research, there are also problems of quality because of poor research design, faulty indexing (McDonald, Lefebvre and Clarke, 1996) and even fraud (Lock, 1988). Additionally there are problems of publication delay (Stern and Simes, 1997) and bias. A 20-year review of four major medical journals in the United States showed that research done in the USA has the best chance of being selected for publication, followed by work from other English-speaking countries (Day, 1997). There is no evidence to suggest

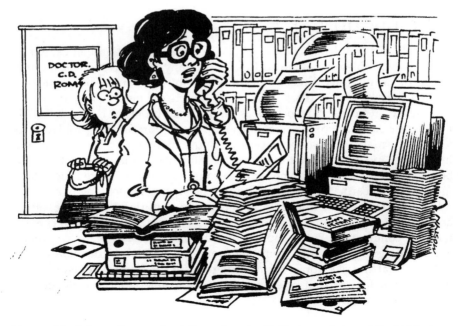

Figure 4.1 Information overload. Reproduced with kind permission of David Mostyn.

that other subjects or other journals are very different. There is similar prejudice against the publication of negative results (Esterbrook *et al.*, 1991).

As well as having to take account of the problems generated before, and during, the process of publication, the beleaguered health professional must also grapple with organisational and personal factors. Personal preference and style can affect information retrieval as much as the way in which information is stored and managed. Lack of time, perceived information overload and lack of skills in using both printed and electronic resources are all factors that contribute to unsystematic methods of information retrieval. When coupled with inefficient information management systems, poor organisation of resources, or underresourced inaccessible libraries, the practitioner may well consider that 'finding the evidence' represents an insurmountable obstacle (Figure 4.1).

Personal factors

In teaching people how to use information systems it is often assumed that information is a discrete, even concrete, reality; that it is a commodity to be acquired. However, information seekers are not 'empty buckets', but individuals who not only collect, store, retrieve and use information, but also create it; moreover they appear to behave differently towards information in different situations and at different times (Dervin, 1977).

Information seeking is affected by characteristics of the information itself, of the receiver, of the task, of the organisation and of the environment (Brown, 1983). Information is not intrinsic to the data. The information sought will also vary with the stage reached by the seeker in the process of problem solution. There are, of course, many different kinds of problems, each demanding a different strategy for its solution (Childs, 1986, p. 172):

> there are circumstances in which the same person will tackle similar problems in different ways – these are situation specific strategies. But, by and large, in each person patterns are established ('response sets') which are compounded to give individuality to learning and problem-solving processes.

Several general types of strategy, or extended sequences of behaviour, have been described; one of the most pervasive is confirmation bias. Research in perception has shown that expectation often determines what is perceived. People shown red spades on playing cards exhibit denial and fixation (Kuhn, 1970). When given a reasoning task, they repeatedly failed to test their hypotheses adequately, and typically engaged in confirmation (Wason, 1960). However, hypothesis-confirmation strategies are sensible if cognitive efficiency is taken into account, since fewer information-processing steps are involved (Skov and Sherman, 1986). Less sensible, and observed as frequently, was the tendency Mahoney found to ask questions about features that had extreme values for the hypothesis in question so that 'subjects will see their hypotheses confirmed more often than they are in fact true.' Apart from confirmation bias, Mahoney recorded an impressive array of 'selective perception, distortion, confirmatory bias, selective recall, and so on, all [of which] seem to conspire toward the protection and maintenance of prior beliefs' (Mahoney, 1979, p. 356).

There have also been many investigations of cognitive style. Style is concerned with manner rather than effectiveness or level of performance, and has been found to be stable over a broad range of applications. It is commonly bipolar and value free, thus distinguishing it from ability dimensions such as intelligence (Messick, 1976). One of the earliest descriptions of cognitive style resulted from Witkin's work on field dependence and independence (Witkin, Moore and Goodenough, 1977). Other classifications include Kirton's Adaption–Innovation theory, in which he proposed a continuum of cognitive style with the ends labelled adaptive (doing things better) and innovative (doing things differently) (Kirton, 1976) and Hudson's classification of schoolboys as divergers or convergers (Hudson, 1966). Learners have also been classified by Pask and Scott (1976) as 'holists' or global learners and 'serialists' or step-by-step learners. Many investigations of learning style have used either Kolb and Fry's (1975) Learning Style Inventory, which classifies learners as convergers, divergers, assimilators or accommodators, or the Learning Style Questionnaire developed later by Honey and Mumford (1992), which distinguishes activists, reflectors, theorists and pragmatists. How preferred learning styles affect educational processes as well as information-seeking behaviour has been the focus of several studies (Ford, 1985; Ford and Ford, 1993; Worth and Fidler, 1997).

Understanding how preferred cognitive style and organisational constraints can affect effective information retrieval is important if the development of new evidence-based information sources, and recommended strategies for coping with the biomedical literature, are to have maximum impact on changing the way in which people reach decisions.

INFORMATION, PROBLEM SOLVING AND EVIDENCE-BASED PRACTICE

Problem finding, hypothesis formation, hypothesis testing and problem solving are integral to the process of clinical practice and research, as is information processing. The similarities of all these processes can be seen by comparing models of problem-solving information processing and the practice of evidence-based medicine. In a typical model of problem solving, Gordon (1974) proposed the following steps:

1. Identify the problem
2. Generate alternative solutions
3. Evaluate alternatives
4. Choose a solution

5. Implement the solution
6. Evaluate the results.

These steps are very similar to models of information processing and information transfer which include the stages of idea generation, question formulation, analysis, interpretation, evaluation, organisation, synthesis, repackaging, dissemination and retrieval (Browne, 1997).

The common elements of both the models above are further reflected in the model for evidence-based medicine proposed by Sackett et al (1997), who specify the following necessary stages:

1. Translation of the problem to an answerable question
2. Efficient tracking down of the best external evidence
3. Critical appraisal of the evidence for its validity and clinical applicability
4. Application of the results of the critical appraisal in clinical practice
5. Evaluation of one's performance.

However, evidence-based healthcare is much more than a technique for processing information or solving problems because it emphasises that the best external evidence must be integrated with individual clinical expertise and the patient's choice in a bottom-up approach. It further stresses that external clinical evidence can inform, but can never replace, individual clinical expertise.

FINDING THE EVIDENCE

Finding relevant and high-quality information to inform healthcare decisions can represent a daunting task for many health professionals. Typically, a search may include data from personal experience, observation, research and laboratory results, or published and unpublished studies. In the next sections we look at:

- the varieties of published information and their usefulness for evidence-based practitioners
- a structured approach to searching databases
- methods for the management and storage of information.

Sources of evidence

The growth of an evidence-based culture has resulted in the development of new information sources that aim to eliminate the difficulties inherent in existing sources. However, for many healthcare questions the traditional literature remains the only source for reference. It is important, therefore, to recognise the limitations of such traditional sources and also to keep abreast of the development of new specialised sources for evidence-based healthcare. Before going on to describe the range of information sources available, it is useful to identify and reflect on what you currently do when you need to find information on effectiveness (Box 4.1).

Books

Reference books, which include dictionaries, encyclopaedias, directories and handbooks, are usually consulted for single pieces of information. They need to be revised regularly as the information they hold goes out of date quickly. Textbooks, or monographs, are an important source of core knowledge and offer a standard account of a subject. However, they also become out of date quickly, and the time taken to publish new editions means that they are partly out of date as soon as they are published. Also, as Williams, Baker and Marshall (1992) have suggested, books tend to be opinion based rather than evidence based, and should not be relied on as a sole source. Other forms of printed publication include reports, theses and 'grey' literature. Reports are produced regularly by government departments, professional bodies, universities, and other statutory and voluntary organisations. Grey literature is documentation produced on an *ad hoc* basis either locally or nationally which is not formally published, for example local health surveys, policy statements, codes of practice, research studies and project reports.

Journals

These may also be known as serials or periodicals and are publications issued at regular intervals. Journals contain primary reports of investigations or research and are more current, although delays may still occur between writing and publication. The articles in most reputable scientific

---

Box **4.1** Where do you go to find information?

1. When did you last need information?
2. What sources did you use to satisfy your query? Information sources need not be confined to textbooks and journals. You might have used printed sources, electronic sources, the knowledge of colleagues or your own experience.
3. List these sources on a piece of paper.
4. Try to identify the advantages and disadvantages for each source.
5. Think about the factors that led you to choose these sources (e.g. ease of access, quality of the source, previous experience).
6. Finally, how might your search for information have been facilitated?

journals are peer reviewed, a process that involves the articles being sent to 'expert' reviewers before being accepted for publication. Printed indexes and abstract publications can be used to find journal articles. These secondary sources provide references to the contents of the primary journals and can be searched via author and subject, within a range of specified titles. Many of these indexing and abstracting tools are now available in electronic format as computer databases.

Databases

Unlike printed indexes, electronic databases allow a search to be carried out for a combination of subjects and authors, across a range of years. Databases such as MEDLINE, CINAHL and EMBASE (see Box 4.2) mirror the structure of a printed index. In contrast, the Cochrane Library, rather than providing references to single articles in primary journals, synthesises the results of many primary published and unpublished studies in structured systematic reviews.

There are many ways to access the same data. For example, the MEDLINE database produced by the National Library of Medicine in the United States can be accessed:

- on-line through a commercial host such as Datastar or Dialog
- on CD-ROM from a commercial supplier such as OVID Technologies or SilverPlatter
- via the Internet
- via a professional organisation such as the British Medical Association
- in print form using *Index Medicus.*

Although the search software and access routes are different, the data are the same.

Box **4.2** Bibliographical databases

The following list of databases does not seek to be comprehensive, but includes the major bibliographical databases currently available which index healthcare information.

ASSIA The database has a strong emphasis on applied aspects of the social sciences. Key subject fields covered include sociology, psychology, cultural anthropology, politics and economics (Coverage: 1987 to date).

CANCERLIT The database covers the treatment of cancer as well as information on epidemiology, pathogenesis and immunology (Coverage: 1963 to date).

Box 4.2 Cont'd

CINAHL The nursing and allied health database covers all aspects of nursing and allied health disciplines such as health education, occupational therapy, emergency services, social services in health care (Coverage: 1983 to date).

DHSS-DATA Department of Health database covering key fields of health service and hospital administration, medical equipment and supplies, public health, nursing, primary care, social policy and social services. Approximately 40% of records have abstracts (Coverage: 1983 to date). *Note:* Although the database is updated weekly, indexing is slow and the currency of information may be a problem.

EMBASE European equivalent of MEDLINE, the *Excerpta Medica* database is a good source for drug and pharmacology information, over 40% of entries being drug related. Other aspects of human medicine covered include health policy, drug and alcohol dependence, psychiatry, forensic science and pollution control. Worldwide coverage with a European focus (Coverage: 1974 to date).

HEALTH-CD A new database (April 1997) produced by The Stationery Office which has the full text of many publications and documents from the Department of Health. The database is split into three sections: main collection, Acts of Parliament and statutory instruments.

HealthSTAR This database (formerly known as HealthPlan) covers the literature on the non-clinical aspects of healthcare delivery, including all aspects of administration and planning of healthcare facilities, evaluation of patient outcomes, effectiveness of procedures, health technology, health insurance and financial management, personnel management, staff deployment and quality assurance (Coverage: 1975 to date).

MEDLINE The US National Library of Medicine's bibliographical database covers the whole field of medical information and is the most widely used database of its type in the world. Abstracts are available for 70% of entries (Coverage: 1966 to date).

PsychLIT Contains summaries of the world's serial literature in psychology and related disciplines and is compiled from the PsychInfo database. PsychLIT covers 1300 journals in 27 languages from approximately 50 countries. PsychLIT also has a chapters and books section to the database, which contains summaries of English

Box **4.2** Cont'd

language chapters and books in psychology and related disciplines published worldwide. To integrate behavioural information from other fields, publications are scanned from related disciplines, such as sociology, linguistics, medicine, law, physiology, business, psychiatry and anthropology (Coverage: journal articles from 1974 to date; chapters and books from 1987 to date).

SIGLE   The System for Information on Grey Literature in Europe is produced by the European Association for Grey Literature Exploitation. Grey literature is best defined as literature that cannot readily be acquired through normal bookselling channels and which is therefore difficult to identify or obtain (Coverage: 1980 to date).

New sources for evidence-based healthcare

The ability to find evidence systematically about clinical effectiveness, especially in reviews and other summaries, is a key skill for the evidence-based practitioner. To use these resources effectively, healthcare professionals need to acquire knowledge and skills: knowledge about the range, quality and content of available sources of evidence about effectiveness, irrespective of format, and skills to use these sources effectively.

Evidence on clinical effectiveness can be found in newsletters and bulletins, such as the *Effective Health Care* series produced by the National Health Service (NHS) Centre for Reviews and Dissemination in York, and *Bandolier*, a newsletter designed to keep health professionals up to date with both local and national initiatives and literature on the effectiveness of healthcare interventions.

Primary journals, as we have described them, should be distinguished from a new type of secondary journal which provides detailed abstracts from published studies and reviews. These journals, for example *ACP Journal Club* and *Evidence-based Medicine, Evidence-based Nursing, Evidence-based Health Policy and Management,* only choose articles that meet strict selection criteria. Each article is summarised in a structured abstract, with an expert commentary that sets the information in a clinical perspective.

The Cochrane Library is the primary source for retrieving high-quality evidence in the form of systematic reviews and is the product of the Cochrane Collaboration, an international network of individuals committed to preparing, maintaining, and disseminating systematic, up-to-date reviews of the effects of health care. It includes the following databases:

1. The Cochrane Database of Systematic Reviews (CDSR) (now searchable on the web) is a rapidly growing collection of regularly updated systematic reviews of the effects of healthcare.

2. The York Database of Abstracts of Reviews of Effectiveness (DARE) provides structured abstracts of published systematic reviews. These include good-quality reviews that have been quality filtered by reviewers at the NHS Centre for Reviews and Dissemination, as well as briefer records of reviews that may be useful for background information. Abstracts of reports of health technology agencies worldwide have now been included, as have abstracts of reviews produced by the American College of Physician's Journal Club up to 1995.

3. The Cochrane Controlled Trials Register (CCTR) is a bibliography of over 150, 000 controlled trials, including many not currently listed in MEDLINE or other bibliographical databases. (Full version available only on the CD-ROM version of the Cochrane Library.)

4. The Cochrane Review Methodology Database (CRMD) is a bibliography of articles on the science of research synthesis and on practical aspects of preparing systematic reviews.

Another useful source is Best Evidence, a CD-ROM which contains the full text of two major journals of secondary publication: *ACP Journal Club* and *Evidence-Based Medicine*. Both journals cover reviews from more than 90 journals worldwide, and choose only those articles that meet strict selection criteria for study design. Each article is summarised in a structured abstract, with expert commentary putting the information in clinical context.

Many traditional and new sources are becoming accessible via the Internet. Over the past 3 years the Internet has grown in importance as a source of healthcare information. In spite of all the hyperbole, the experience of many users is of unreliable connections, slow access, problems in identifying information and a general difficulty in finding anything useful in what has been called a 'giant data heap' (Robinson and Bawden, 1995). For health professionals in the NHS there are added difficulties. Unlike their colleagues in the higher education sector who have enjoyed access to many facilities through the Joint Academic Network (JANET) for many years, in the NHS the experience of accessing networked information is far from a daily reality. Even when all Trusts and health authorities are connected to the NHS net, the difficulties of accessing high-quality information for evidence-based healthcare will remain. However, there are an increasing number of guides to sources and sites on the Internet.

Two of the most reliable sources are Netting the Evidence (http://www.shef.ac.uk/uni/academic/R-Z/scharr/ir/netting.html) produced by the Sheffield Centre for Health and Related Research (ScHARR) and the OMNI (Organising Medical Networked Information) Gateway (http://www.omni.ac.uk). The URLs (Uniform Resource Locators) for these sites are given in brackets. Detailed lists of other Internet addresses have not been given, as they may change frequently. More information on useful sources of evidence can be found via the sites mentioned above, or from your local health library.

STRUCTURED APPROACHES TO SEARCHING FOR EVIDENCE

As we have seen, evidence-based healthcare requires access to an increasing number of information resources, including databases, primary and secondary journals, reports and grey literature. With the proliferation of personal computers, modems, CD-ROMs, local area networks and the growth of the Internet, many practitioners are accustomed to searching databases for 'one or two relevant articles'. However, to extract high-quality evidence from a database it is necessary to understand some of the idiosyncrasies of database searching and how search techniques can dramatically affect outcomes.

The need for information skills training is well recognised. Many of the relevant issues have been and are being addressed in the NHS Training Division's education and training programme in Information Management and Technology (IM&T) for clinicians, in the higher education Electronic Libraries Programme (eLib), and in many local and regional initiatives. In Oxford, for example, the development of Finding the Evidence Workshops (Palmer, 1996) to train a broad spectrum of health professionals in information skills developed out of a need expressed by participants attending workshops in critical appraisal in the Critical Appraisal Skills Programme (http://wwwlib.jr2.ox.ac.uk/caspfew/).

In the following section we look at some of the factors that contribute to a successful search.

Asking the question

Models of problem solving, information seeking and evidence-based healthcare all agree on the critical importance of question formulation not only in information searching but also in clinical practice (Richardson *et al.*, 1995; Flemming, 1998). Indeed, Richardson *et al.* (1995) suggest that it is helpful to phrase the question to facilitate searching. For clinicians, any encounter with a patient may elicit a question. By formulating the clinical problem in terms of the patient or condition, the intervention or exposure being considered and the clinical outcome, a 'well-built clinical question' is constructed that helps to identify knowledge gaps and indicate where the information need exists. For clinicians and information professionals, the task of analysing the question in this way enables a clearer understanding of how the component concepts relate to one another and enables a more structured search for information. Creating a grid to record the process is helpful. For example, a common problem is to assess the risks (outcome) in treating or not treating (intervention) a given condition (condition) for a particular patient or group of patients (patient) (see Table 4.1).

Table 4.1		
Patient/Condition	**Intervention**	**Outcome**
	Treatment	Risk Factors
	No Treatment	
	Drug Therapy	

Search terms

Once clarified, the question must be amplified by drawing up a list of synonyms or similar words that may also lead to the desired information source. These 'natural language' terms, or 'free text' terms as they are sometimes called, can be used for searching on any database. If the searcher does not specify what part of the record is to be searched, the search software will default to the entire record. An exact match will be found for whatever character strings are entered – often with unexpected and sometimes entertaining results. A search for the term 'BRAIN' will pick up a match for that string of characters as author, as a title word and as a word in the abstract. Because a literal match of characters is made, plurals, grammatical variants and alternative spellings will not be retrieved; for example, entering the word pregnancy will not retrieve pregnant or pregnancies. Similarly, preterm birth will not retrieve premature birth (synonyms), and diarrhoea will not retrieve diarrhea (English and American spellings). Most databases build in some search techniques to overcome this problem; for example, the use of a symbol (* on WinSpirs, $ on Ovid), known as a truncation symbol, at the end of a word will include any number of further characters, or the wild card (? on WinSpirs) in the middle of a word will replace one or no letters. So, on WinSpirs, diarrh* will retrieve diarrhoea or diarrhea, or diarrhoeal or diarrheal, etc., and an?emia will retrieve anemia or anaemia.

Understanding and using Medical Subject Headings

Natural language terms are not sufficient for a comprehensive search. All information banks, that is libraries of books or databases of journal references of the web sites on the Internet, provide 'finding tools' for the information seeker in the shape of indexes and catalogues. Typically, these use a controlled alphabetical or hierarchical list of preferred and related terms to channel and limit the information search. For example, in healthcare, the National Library of Medicine has developed the Medical Subject Headings (MeSH) list which specifies terms to be used by their indexers in compiling entries for the MEDLINE database. There is a similar list for indexers compiling entries for the Cumulated Index for Nursing and Allied Health

(CINAHL) and most other databases. Thus, for example, KIDNEY DISEASES is preferred to RENAL DISEASES. The electronic forms of MEDLINE and CINAHL (Ovid Technology and SilverPlatter) have a built-in list of index terms called a thesaurus. When using the SilverPlatter version, the system will assume that that you are using 'natural language' terms, whereas with the Ovid Technology's version the system assumes that the search terms are derived from the thesaurus.

What are the advantages of using these so-called 'preferred terms' when searching on databases? The use of preferred subject headings and index-ing terms allows the grouping together of information sources that may not contain indicative or relevant words in the title or abstract and which would otherwise be difficult to find if only 'natural language' terms were used. Thus an article or book may be about breast cancer, and indexed as such, but may not include those exact words in the title or abstract. It is important to realise that, while references may be retrieved using 'natural language terms', these are unlikely to represent the complete set of refer-ences present in the database. The use of natural language terms together with index terms is more likely to lead to a thorough search.

Thus a search of MEDLINE (1990–1996) reveals a significant difference in references retrieved:

thrush (natural language)   retrieves 157
candidiasis, oral (MeSH)   retrieves 687

However, these index 'languages' impose a requirement on the searcher to translate the question in terms of the predetermined list of subject words. The idiosyncrasies of indexes and thesauri can be frustrating and even intimidating for the searcher. Further, indexing practice may prescribe that indexers assign the most specific index term, whereas a searcher may assume the reverse, namely that all articles are indexed according to the broadest term. For example, in the case of cancer, MEDLINE and CINAHL indexers are instructed to index articles in the most specific way. An article about breast cancer will not be indexed under cancer, nor under the preferred term NEOPLASMS, but rather under the specific term BREAST NEOPLASMS.

It is important to appreciate the way in which articles are indexed and some of the helpful built-in features that exist. For most MeSH terms there will be broader, narrower and related terms to consider for selection within the thesaurus contained in the database. A good way to find what index-ing terms are used is to type in 'natural language' word(s) and, having retrieved some references, to browse through a few records, paying particular attention to the MeSH field, located just below the abstract, which contains the Medical Subject Headings. These index terms can suggest additional MeSH terms, which can then be used with the natural language terms that have already been selected.

Search strategies

To make sure that the search is not inadvertently limited and as many papers as possible are included at the beginning, it is useful to use the facility for 'explosion' in searching. When a thesaurus term (in MEDLINE or CINAHL) is 'exploded', all the articles that have been indexed as narrower (more specific) terms, and which are listed below the broader (more general) term, will be included automatically. For example, 'exploding' INTESTINAL NEOPLASMS would find papers indexed not only under this term but also articles on neoplasms associated with more specific parts of the intestine such as COLONIC NEOPLASMS, DUODENAL NEOPLASMS, etc. and indexed under these terms.

It is also possible to use subheadings, such as -diagnosis, -contra-indications, -therapy, etc. in association with index terms, but it is important to recognise that the use of these will refine the search. It is also useful for the searcher to understand that, because entries are compiled by human beings, the quality of the database might be flawed. This is true even of well-regarded, high-quality databases such as MEDLINE. Thus work carried out by the UK Cochrane Centre has shown that, even though an article may be reporting a randomised control trial, the indexers may fail to use this term in indexing the entry. This underlines the importance of developing a search strategy which uses both natural language and indexing terms.

'Natural language' words and index or thesauri terms can be combined in a search 'strategy' with the Boolean operators, AND and OR. The use of these operators can be illustrated with a very simple example: combining the search terms dogs and cats with OR will yield all the references that are about dogs as well as all the references that are about cats (the mnemonic 'OR is more' is helpful). Using the operator AND, on the other hand, will yield only those papers that happen to be about dogs and cats, and will exclude those that are about only dogs or only cats.

Sensitivity, specificity and the quality of the evidence

A sound search strategy therefore begins by extracting as many references as possible (a sensitive search) and then moves on to defining the requirement more precisely (a specific search). Once a comprehensive set of references has been created, the task of looking within this set for high-quality material may begin. (See Chapters 2 and 3 for a description of levels of evidence, and the relevance of different types of study in answering different types of questions.) Researchers at the McMaster Health Information Research Unit and the UK Cochrane Centre call this process 'panning for gold'. They have developed a special set of search strategies, called quality filters, which may include a few or many search terms, to increase the effectiveness of the search by retrieving the most appropriate studies. For example, in looking for articles about therapeutic interventions, the recommended quality filter to use (from 1990) is CLINICAL TRIAL as a publication type (pt). Before 1990 the recommended term to use is RANDOM* as a natural language term. The 'publication type' field was introduced in 1991 to complement main headings. It indicates what type of publication is being indexed, rather than what the publication is about.

This highlights the importance of recognising that indexing practice changes over the years and that it may be necessary to check what MeSH terms might have been used previously. There is also a recommended quality filter for retrieving reviews (including overviews and meta-analyses) in MEDLINE (McKibbon *et al.*, 1996).

These methodological search filters can help you retrieve sound clinical studies that deal with diagnosis, prognosis, therapy, aetiology, guidelines, treatment outcomes and evidence-based healthcare methods. They can be added to your subject search and provide a reliable method for finding high-quality evidence quickly (these can be viewed and downloaded at http://www.ihs.ox.ac.uk/library/filters.html).

OBTAINING THE EVIDENCE

Once appropriate and useful references have been identified in a search, the next step is to obtain these articles, reviews or books. This can be the hardest part of sourcing your information need. For many healthcare professionals in the NHS there are no automatic rights of access to a healthcare library and, where access is available, this is often only during the working day (Fennessy, 1997). Even when access is unproblematic, the process of borrowing a book, or obtaining a copy of the full article from a scientific journal, can seem unreasonably slow, especially when the search may have been conducted swiftly on an electronic database and when so much information is apparently immediately obtainable on the Internet.

Where there is a local or professional health library, this can supply almost any document from a wide variety of sources. Librarians call this process 'document delivery' whether it involves books, reports or photocopied articles. As electronic publishing and the Internet impact on methods of document supply, there has been a noticeable shift towards providing access to sources when needed ('just in time'), rather than stockpiling large collections of journals 'just in case'. The format and media in which a document has been published will determine the best method of obtaining it.

Library and information services will provide the required material either from their own stock or through interlibrary lending schemes.

The library's own stock

There will normally be access to a wide range of information resources, including books, current journals and newspapers. Photocopiers will be provided for self-service photocopying, although some photocopying may be done on behalf of readers by library staff. The library's own catalogue, usually held on a computer, will record all items held in stock. The catalogue may also include journals, annual reports and theses, and will usually allow a search to be made by subject or author. Most health libraries order their material using one of many classification schemes, such as that developed by the National Library of Medicine. Once located, documents may be either loaned or copied, subject to the provisions of the Copyright, Designs and Patents Act 1988 (see Box 4.3).

Interlibrary lending

The absence of a desired item in any one library does not mean that the item is unobtainable. Libraries extend the resources that are available to readers many times over through cooperative schemes. Many healthcare libraries participate in regional interlending schemes whereby, on payment of a token or charge, a photocopy or loan can be obtained for a reader, again subject to the provisions of the Copyright Act. For a summary of these regulations, see Box 4.3. Beyond the confines of a particular Region, there are other sources and other networks. There are also national schemes, run on a commercial footing, such as that operated by the British Library Document Supply Centre, or those offered by the libraries of professional bodies such as the British Medical Association or Royal College of Nursing (there will also usually be a fee for this service). Copyright is a complex issue. The need to comply with legislation imposes certain procedures. These may often appear to library users to be needlessly bureaucratic and even obstructive when they are required to sign forms and are denied multiple copies of articles. It is important for all clinicians to be aware of the requirements of the Act.

Box **4.3** Copyright

What follows is an attempt to summarise what is permissible under the legislation. Further guidance can be obtained from your local health library or from the publications listed at the end of this chapter.

The Copyright, Designs and Patents Act 1988 restricts the amount of material that can be copied from published works without either the permission of the copyright owner or a licence. Infringement may lead to prosecution, and substantial fines may be imposed.

Box **4.3** Cont'd

PRINTED MATERIAL

There is a difference between what library staff may copy on your behalf and what you may copy for yourself.

Self-service photocopying

The Act permits individuals to make copies of parts of printed material such as books, journals, newspapers and indexes under 'fair dealing', provided that the copies are for research or private study and do not constitute a 'substantial' part of the work. Copies should be marked with source details, both as acknowledgement and for future quotation.

Photocopying by library staff

There is a specific set of regulations outlining what library staff may copy for a reader. The main points are:

- The reader must sign a copyright declaration form for each item requested.
- A charge must be made for copies made by library staff.

For the main types of publication, the restrictions specified are as follows.

Journals

Library staff may supply only one copy of a single article from any single issue of a journal at any one time to a reader.
Note: Readers able to visit the library who require more than one article from a single issue may be able to make such copies for themselves under 'fair dealing' as outlined above. Alternatively, library staff may be able to fulfil such requests through the British Library copyright cleared service, provided that the British Library Document Supply Centre is satisfied the customer is not using the service as a substitute for purchase. This service currently costs approximately 25% more than the standard charge. Further details can be obtained from your local health library.

Books and reports

Library staff may not copy more than a 'reasonable proportion' of a book. As a guideline, this can be defined as no more than 5% of the total book or one complete chapter.

Box 4.3 Cont'd

HMSO publications

HMSO will allow one copy of the whole item, provided it is for one individual in an organisation, and that copies are not distributed to other individuals or organisations. Multiple copies can be made of extracts up to 30% of the entire work, or one complete chapter (even if this is more than 30%) from specified categories of material.
 Other priced HMSO publications may not contain any information about copyright and photocopying. However, the normal regulations covering books and journals may still apply, and normal restrictions apply unless permission has been given.

Non-HMSO government publications

Department of Health publications and circulars may be copied in full. If there are any doubts, contact the Department of Health. Other non-HMSO government publications often do not contain any information about copyright and photocopying. However, the normal regulations covering books and journals may still apply, and normal restrictions apply unless permission has been given.

ON-LINE AND CD-ROM DATABASES

Databases accessed via on-line hosts or CD-ROM have their own licensing terms which are available from the host/supplier. These will detail how much data can be downloaded and in what format. An example of the restrictions on MEDLINE on the SilverPlatter CD-ROM database is given below:

... the customer is ... granted ... licence to:

a) *make searches on the database*
b) *make one or more copies of any search output in hard copy form, which may be utilised by the customer, but may not be sold*
c) *make copies of any search output in electronic form i.e. diskette, hard disk or tape – to be used for editing or temporary storage only*
d) *make one copy of the software diskette and documentation for archival purposes only.*

See also futher reading on p.83

Electronic document delivery

Technology is altering our concept of what a 'document' means and raising the expectations of all professionals for instant access to everything from the desktop. For writers, readers, publishers and librarians the problems posed by electronic publishing are complex and manifold, and include, for example, cost, copyright and the impact on scholarly communication. However, in practical terms, for most people, electronic document delivery (EDD) means downloading a list of references or the full text of a document from databases or full-text sources (e.g. on CD-ROM or the Internet).

An increasing number of books and journals are becoming available electronically in full text. These are being marketed on either a subscription or a pay-as-you-go basis by a wide range of commercial providers, including publishers, providers of on-line databases and other suppliers. Some on-line providers are also providing links from bibliographical databases such as MEDLINE, directly to the full text of documents. Many of these services are offered via the Internet and the World Wide Web using popular browsers such as Netscape and Internet Explorer. Full texts are either held on the provider's server or accessed via a gateway on the publisher's own server. These services allow access to full-text articles by authorised subscribers, searching of the table of contents in journals and abstracts. Some services are targeted at groups of professionals and include related services such as bulletin boards, current awareness and discussion groups. Any user of these services will need to assess and compare providers in what is a highly changeable and volatile market.

New developments in EDD

Within the higher education sector there have been a series of initiatives arising from the Follett Review of university libraries in 1993. Two of the most important of these have been the Pilot Site Licence Initiative, which has sought to provide access to electronic versions of journals for users of academic libraries, and the Electronic Libraries (eLib) Programme which, with a budget of over £15 million has funded 60 projects over the past 3 years. Amongst the many issues associated with electronic libraries, eLib has included a number of projects that have focused on the development of models to promote and improve effective retrieval of documents through electronic means.

These include the Joint Electronic Document Delivery Software (JEDDS) project and the LAMDA (London and Manchester Document Access) project. An interesting aspect of both these projects is that they use Ariel, a software package that is a document transmission system made and developed by the Research Libraries Group, USA, which promises faster, more reliable, transmission. Ariel allows users to scan articles, photos and similar documents, transmit the resulting electronic images over the Internet to another Ariel workstation, or e-mail them to properly equipped e-mail accounts, and print theses. The system, which is optimised for Internet transmission, is less expensive to use than facsimile transmission and produces images of greater resolution and quality. Ariel is not a document delivery service itself. It is simply a tool that libraries, document delivery services and other sources use to deliver documents. The actual documents that can be received via Ariel depend on what can be supplied by document suppliers or the offices using Ariel themselves.

The theme of the second phase of the Electronic Libraries Programme which has just begun is 'Building Models for the Future of the Library'. The new programme will find model ways to integrate print and electronics content in the so-called 'hybrid library'.

Another project, SEREN (Sharing Educational Resources in an Electronic Network in Wales) has linked together all the educational establishments that come under the umbrella of the University of Wales to produce a database of bibliographical holdings for them. This is then used to provide a fast and effective interlibrary lending service. The user (currently the librarian, but soon to be the end-user) searches for the required article, picks a location that holds it and sends off a request by e-mail. At the other end, a receipt station processes the request. The article is then scanned in and sent off to the user. When received, it prompts the user for a signed copyright form and payment.

Many issues have to be addressed before the aim of a cost-effective, multiple scenario, user-friendly EDD system is achieved. The requirements for such a service do not yet exist. There would need to be standard protocols, consistent software, access to a wide range of services, protection of intellectual copyright and adequate funding. There would also have to be support for viewing and printing formats, support of e-mail standards, a minimum workstation specification, printing services and managed accounts and passwords.

STORING THE EVIDENCE

Many health professionals assiduously collect photocopied articles, copies of books, reports and other printed materials, and place these on shelves, in filing cabinets, on the desk and even the floor. As the quantity increases, so the task of organising the content becomes more daunting and the likelihood of retrieving the contents more remote. How this personal collection of evidence might be managed for efficient later retrieval is seldom considered. Effective practice requires an equally effective mechanism for the storage of evidence if the contents are to be retrieved later. Computer-based text retrieval systems allow much easier access to personal collections and also allow retrieval from different entry points.

Personal Bibliographic Software (PBS)

PBS is a class of text retrieval software designed to enable users to manage their personal reference collections. What differentiates PBS from the many other types of database software is the extent to which it is specialised to deal with bibliographical references (Hanson, 1995). It provides a mechanism for creating a reference database as well as bibliographies for the use of an organisation or individual.

These software packages are generally user-friendly and easy to use. Predefined data structures with sophisticated search capabilities allow the user to import information from on-line and CD-ROM databases. There are also predefined output formats which enable citations to be written easily in a variety of style conventions (e.g. Harvard, Vancouver), and subject bibliographies can be produced quickly.

One of the advantages of using PBS is that importing data is much faster and easier than typing in references, or writing out index cards, offering fast and efficient retrieval similar to searching CD-ROM databases. As with all software packages, effective use requires training and access to technical support. Back-ups will have to be made and upgrades obtained when required.

Choosing a PBS package is a personal decision and several factors need to be taken into consideration in order to evaluate, select and support an appropriate solution (Nicholl *et al.*, 1996). These include perceived uses and needs for the package, system requirements, support and training, cost, local or organisational preferences, and flexibility. Search capabilities are important, as is compatibility with word-processing packages and database integrity. It is important to ascertain whether the package allows electronic importation from the sources you most use (e.g. bibliographical databases).

There are now many interesting Internet sites which link to pages of interest on PBS. Some contain mainly sales material, some provide demonstrations, and some provide evaluations and summaries on the functions of particular software packages. Used carefully these sites can provide useful information, as well as provide links to other sites of interest.

THE GOAL OF EVIDENCE-BASED PRACTICE

The practice of evidence-based healthcare imposes certain requirements. These can be simply summarised as:

- *Awareness* of the range of sources and of their uses and limitations
- *Access* to libraries and information services and to the skills of an expert information specialist
- *Connection* to networked information services either on local area networks or on the Internet
- *Competence* in searching for information through training.

In this chapter we have outlined the skills and sources necessary for effective practice. The best way to improve knowledge and skills is through practice and with the help of local health librarians. However, it is important to recognise that, however willing individuals may be to change their practice, in many circumstances organisational and political constraints exist which appear to undermine these endeavours. If evidence-based practice is to become a reality all professional groups must work together to achieve this end.

REFERENCES

Brown, C.G. (1983). Measures and models to assess the impact of information on complex problem-solving. In *Information Science in Action*, vol. 2, ed. Debons, A. pp. 629–639. The Hague: Martinus Nijhoff.

Browne, M. (1997). The field of information policy 1. Fundamental concepts. *Journal of Information Science*, **23**, 261–275.

Childs, D. (1986). Cognitive styles. In *Personality, Cognition and Values*, ed. Bagley, C. & Verma, G.K. pp. 171–195. London: Macmillan.

Day, M. (1997). The price of prejudice. *New Scientist* **156**, 22–23.

Dervin, B. (1977). Useful theory for librarianship. Communication not information. *Drexel Library Bulletin*, **13**(5), 16–32.

Esterbrook, P.A., Berlin, J.A, Gopalan, R. & Matthews, D.R. (1991). Publication bias in clinical research. *Lancet*, **337**, 867–872.

Fennessy, G. (1997). Qualified nurses losing out. *Nursing Standard*, **12**(6), 26–27.

Flemming, K. (1998). Asking answerable questions. *Evidence-based Nursing*, **1**(2), 36–37.

Ford, N. (1985). Styles and strategies of processing information. Implications for professional education. *Education for Information*, **3**, 115–132.

Ford, N. & Ford, R. (1993). Towards a cognitive theory of information accessing: an empirical study. *Information Processing and Management*, **29**, 5.

Gordon, T. (1974). *Teacher Effectiveness Training*. New York: McKay.

Hanson, T. (1995). *Bibliographic Software and the Electronic Library*. Hatfield: University of Hertfordshire Press.

Honey, P. & Mumford, A. (1992). *The Manual of Learning Styles*, 3rd edn. Maidenhead: Peter Honey.

Hudson, L. (1966). *Contrary Imaginations*. London: Methuen.

Kirton, M.J. (1976). Adaptors and innovators: a description and a measure. *Journal of Applied Psychology*, **61**, 622–629.

Kolb, D.A. & Fry, R. (1975). Towards an applied theory of experiential learning. In *Theories of Group Processes*, ed. Cooper, C.L. pp. 33–57. London: Wiley.

Kuhn, T.S. (1970). *The Structure of Scientific revolutions*. Chicago: University of Chicago Press.

Lock, S. (1988). Fraud in medicine. *British Medical Journal*, **296**, 376–377.

Lynch, C. (1997). Searching the Internet. *Scientific American*, **276**(3), 44–48.

McDonald, S., Lefebvre, C. & Clarke, M. (1996). Identifying reports of controlled trials in the *BMJ* and the *Lancet*. *British Medical Journal*, **313**, 1116–1117.

McKibbon, K.A., Walker-Dilks, C.J., Wilczynski, N.L. & Haynes, R.B. (1996). Beyond the ACP Journal Club: how to harness MEDLINE for review articles. *ACP Journal Club*, **May–June:** A12–13.

Mahoney, M.J. (1979). The psychology of the scientist: an evaluative review. *Social Studies of Science*, **9**, 349–375.

Martyn, J. (1987). *Literature Searching Habits and Attitudes of Research Scientists*. British Library Research paper 14. London: British Library.

Messick, S. (1976). *Individuality in Learning*. San Fransisco: Jossey Bass.

Nicholl, L.H. *et al.* (1996). Bibliographic database managers: a comparative review, *Computers in Nursing*, **14**(1), 45–56.

Palmer, J. (1996). Where is the evidence? – teaching health professionals how to find the evidence. In *Health Information Management: What Strategies?* Proceedings of the Fifth European Conference of Medical and Health Libraries, Coimbra, 1996, ed. Bakker S. pp. 299–301. Dordrecht: Kluwer.

Pask, G. & Scott, B.C.E. (1976). Learning strategies and individual competence. *International Journal of Man–Machine Studies*, **4**, 217–253.

Price, D.J. deSolla (1963). *Little Science, Big Science.* New York: Columbia University Press.
Richardson, S., Wilson, M.C., Nishikawa, J. & Hayward, R.S.A. (1995). The well-built clinical question: a key to evidence-based decisions. *ACP Journal Club,* November–December: A12–13.
Robinson, L. & Bawden, D. (1995). Internet: the way forward. *Managing Information,* 2(3), 20–22.
Sackett, D.L., Richardson, W.S., Rosenberg, W. & Haynes, R.B. (1997). *Evidence-based Medicine: How to Practice and Teach EBM.* New York: Churchill Livingstone.
Skov, R.B. & Sherman, S.J. (1986). Information gathering processes. *Journal of Experimental Social Psychology,* 22, 93–121.
Stern, J.M. & Simes, R.J. (1997). Publication bias: evidence of delayed publication in a cohort study of clinical research projects. *British Medical Journal,* 315, 640–645.
Wason, P.C. (1960). On the failure to eliminate hypotheses in a conceptual task. *Quarterly Journal of Experimental Psychology,* 12, 129–140.
Williams, R.M., Baker, L.M. & Marshall, J.M. (1992). *Information Searching in Health Care.* Thorofare, New Jersey: SLACK.
Witkin, H.A., Moore, C.A. & Goodenough, D.R. (1977). Field-dependent and field-independent cognitive styles and their educational implications. *Review of Educational Research,* 47, 1–64.
Worth, J. & Fidler, C. (1997). Exploring the effects of learning style on the use of an electronic library system. *Library and Information Research News,* 21(68), 43–46.
Wyatt, J. (1991). Use and sources of medical knowledge. *Lancet,* 338, 1368–1373.

Further reading on copyright issues

Copyright Licensing Agency (CLA) home page http://www.cla.co.uk

Copyright, Designs and Patents Act (1988) London: HMSO.

Cornish, G.P. (1997) *Copyright: Interpreting the Law for Libraries and Archives,* 2nd edn. London: Library Association.

Dworkin, G. & Taylor R.D. (1989) *Blackstone's Guide to the Copyright, Designs and Patents Act 1988.* London: Blackstone Press. (This contains the full text of the Act.)

Library Association (1996) *Copyright in National Health Service Libraries,* 2nd edn. London: Library Association.

Statutory Instrument (1989) *No. 1212: Copyright (Librarians and Archivists) (Copying of Copyright Material) Regulations 1989.* London: HMSO.

Wall, R.A. (1994) *The Aslib Guide to Copyright.* London: Aslib.

2

Section 2

Applying the Evidence

5

Clinical effectiveness

David C. Benton

INTRODUCTION

The first four chapters in this book have provided the reader with sources of evidence. These sources should be seen as providing keys to unlocking a knowledge base that can then be applied to practice. This chapter illustrates how such evidence can be applied within the modern health service. Practical approaches from the perspective of both a service provider and healthcare commissioner will be explored. A clear analysis of the various drivers as well as some of the antecedents for progressing the clinical effectiveness agenda will be presented. This chapter, alongside Chapters 6 and 7, provides a window of opportunity for the exploration of evidence-based care. Clinical effectiveness is not a brand new concept. It is, however, a developing field that requires more widespread understanding by practitioners, managers, patients and the public if maximum benefits for all are to be achieved.

WHAT ARE WE TALKING ABOUT?

It is not an exaggeration to say that even informed practitioners, when discussing issues relating to clinical effectiveness, can often leave less informed colleagues with a series of questions. Perhaps most alarming amongst these is: What are they talking about? It would appear that the imprecise use of language often lies at the heart of this confusion. Terms such as efficacy, efficiency and effectiveness are used interchangeably. Even in everyday usage the tendency to use these words interchangeably – they all mean 'to have an effect' but with different application – can cause problems (Burchfield, 1996). In more clinical usage such imprecise inter-changeability of words by the newcomer to the field may draw scorn by those who often deem themselves more informed and critical observers. Such difficulties can be exacerbated further when additional terms such as cost effectiveness and cost benefit are added. Before exploring the topic of clinical effectiveness in its widest context, it is critical that working definitions of the various terms are stated and the relationship to one another understood.

Effectiveness

In simple terms the effectiveness of a treatment or intervention can be thought of as the treatment's ability or power to cause something to happen. It can be a positive or negative effect and it may or may not have an impact clinically. The effect is, however, observable and measurable.

Efficiency

In a mechanistic way the efficiency of something is the ratio of a system's output to its input. It is possible to have a process or system that is very efficient but which may not be effective. For example, in the mid-1980s the way that hospital efficiency was counted was on the basis of the number of people entering hospital and leaving hospital within a certain time-frame. The more people who left hospital within the time-frame, the more efficient the hospital was deemed to be. However, people did not need to be 'better' on leaving hospital: indeed, deaths and discharges were treated as being similar.

Efficacy

Efficacy is a narrower term and often relates to a specific treatment that has been adopted for a particular purpose and has the ability to produce the desired effect – an efficacious remedy or a drug of known efficacy.

Cost effectiveness

Cost effectiveness is a term commonly used when debating issues relating to the evidence-based care movement. It is a term that originates from econometric analysis and is used when attempting to compare the cost of achieving a unit of effect. This is an important issue since it provides a relatively simple means of quantifying the financial and wider resources implications of delivering a specific outcome of treatment.

Cost benefit

Cost benefit is, however, the term used to compare an intervention's costs and benefits. If the benefits in financial terms were greater than the costs then a cost–benefit analysis would suggest that the treatment is worth doing. Cost–benefit analysis is, however, difficult to conduct since to do so accurately requires measurement of not just direct costs to the health service or the individual but also less tangible costs and benefits to patients and society at large. For example, a direct cost might be the cost of treatment and stay in hospital; however, an indirect benefit to society might be the fact that the individual was then able to return to work and earn a wage rather than require some form of sickness benefit funded from government or employer. Health economists argue that, although such an analysis is difficult, it is essential when resources are scarce or cash is limited as in the case of a state-funded healthcare system. By conducting cost–benefit analysis, decision makers and the public at large will then have information available to them that will enable hard choices to be made – achieving the greatest good for the least cost.

Clinical effectiveness

Having noted the often imprecise usage of terms it is, however, the case that most writers on this subject have tended to adopt the definition of clinical effectiveness offered by the Department of Health (1996a). In this definition it can be seen that many of the concepts – effectiveness, efficiency, efficacy and benefit – are encompassed within the single definition; clinical effectiveness, which is:

The extent to which specific clinical interventions, when deployed in the field for a particular patient or population, do what they are intended to do. That is, maintain or improve health and secure the greatest possible health gain from the resources available.

From this definition, the purpose of the clinical effectiveness initiative is to ensure that decisions about clinical services and care are increasingly driven by evidence of clinical effectiveness and cost effectiveness, coupled with systematic review of the evidence on health outcomes so as to secure the greatest health gain for the resources available. With these points in mind the remainder of this chapter examines how clinical effectiveness can become an integral part of care delivery.

LEVERS FOR CHANGE

There are a large number of potential levers for advancing the issues relating to the clinical effectiveness agenda. Some cluster into specific areas while others stand alone. One method of conducting such analysis is to use the PEST (political, economic, social and technological) framework (Fig. 5.1). This was the starting point for the analysis that follows below.

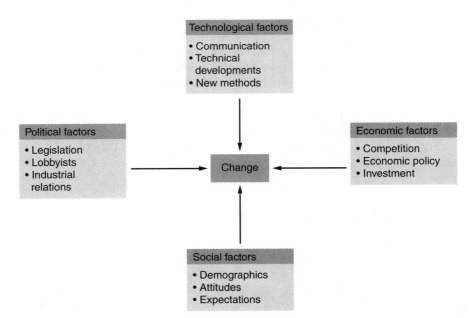

Figure 5.1 An approach to identifying the factors for change.

Resources

The National Health Service (NHS) is a cash-limited publicly funded service. Various changes in the overall population structure, advances in the sophistication of treatments available and the increased expectations of the public have all contributed to escalating demand for service. Whilst modest increases in funding for the health service have been secured to keep pace with general inflation, the inflation associated with healthcare systems tends to run above general inflation. Consequently, year-on-year the health service has had to marshal its resources in such a manner as to meet increased funding pressures. Clinicians of all disciplines are often acutely aware of the need to do more with less. Variously described as cost improvement programmes or efficiency savings, these resource pressures have therefore played a role in driving forward.the clinical effectiveness agenda.

Government policy

As a result of the increased pressure upon resources and a desire to ensure services offered are appropriate in meeting the population needs, year-on-year government policy has accelerated the drive towards the delivery of clinically effective care. Although it could be argued that the best clinical professionals have always striven to advance their practice through clinical audit and other processes, only since the publication of the White Paper *Working for Patients* (Department of Health, 1989), has there been systems-wide pressure to pursue systematic audit. This can perhaps be seen as the antecedence to the current clinical effectiveness policy agenda. Since publication of the White Paper, subsequent government documents such as the annual priority and planning guidance (Department of Health, 1997), various Executive Letters (Department of Health, 1995, 1996b) and subsequent White (Scottish Office Department of Health, 1997) and Green (Scottish Office Department of Health, 1998) Papers published by the health departments have reiterated, reinforced and advanced a focus on delivering clinically effective care.

Public expectations

Increasingly, the public demands more and more information about the various services available to them. Rather than simply leaving it 'to the expert', today's health service user should expect and indeed demand that professionals should furnish them with appropriate information to enable them to make an informed choice. Only when clinicians provide users and potential users of their services with comprehensive, easily understood information, spelling out both advantages and disadvantages, can an informed decision be taken by the client. Both the Patients' Charter (Department of Health, 1991) and the new NHS complaints system (Department of Health, 1996c) have provided additional impetus to the need for the clinical effectiveness of interventions to be shared. Failure to do so can result in increased complaints or, at worst, litigation.

Focused research and development activity

Until relatively recently the health service's research agenda tended to address the particular interests of the scholar or clinician rather than topics that might best inform the coordinated development of services. Michael Peckham, the first NHS Research and Development Director, recognised that this was not the most cost-effective way of spending NHS resources. Accordingly, as a result of changes introduced by him, research and development funding has been targeted towards NHS priority areas. This process identifies gaps in the evidential base and then targets research activity towards these areas, thereby subsequently furnishing clinicians with robust data on the effectiveness of various interventions. The availability of these data on the effectiveness of new interventions can thus shape clinical practice as well as commissioners' priority setting and service investment activities.

It has long been recognised that research studies in themselves often produce conflicting evidence. Clinicians, even those who have some formal research training, can find it difficult to interpret what the totality of research in a particular sphere is in fact saying. Over the past several years, far more meta-analytical studies have been carried out. These studies examine all the available evidence on a particular subject, consider the methodologies used, and attempt to synthesise the results in a way that produces statements akin to a summary of the state of the science. A number of centres have been established to provide a focus for such activity: NHS Centre for Reviews and Dissemination, UK Cochrane Centre, Centre for Evidence Based Nursing, Centre for Evidence Based Medicine, National Centre for Clinical Audit, and the UK Clearing House for Information on the Assessment of Health Outcomes (contact details are given in Appendix 1).

Educational preparation

The move of colleges of nursing into the further and higher education sector is resulting in a change of culture. This new culture is receptive to research and academic scholarship which combines with clinical excellence and teaching to provide an environment supportive of clinically effective care. The net result of this is to develop an educational culture where critical enquiry and evidence-based practice is given much higher priority. In recent years both nursing and professions allied to medicine have upgraded the levels of academic preparation for prequalification programmes to, as a minimum, a higher diploma level. If this is taken alongside the increased numbers of practitioners who are pursuing masters and doctoral degrees, a considerable cadre of clinicians is available and competent to challenge practice in a more robust and scientific manner.

Technology

The introduction of computer technology to the dissemination of information has made major changes in the way that clinicians can access information on clinically effective care. Many hospitals, and indeed wards and departments, have access to the Cumulative Index of Nursing and Allied Health Literature (CINAHL) or MEDLINE-type databases. This facilitates practitioners accessing the most up-to-date information on a particular condition or treatment. Similarly, the increased availability of the Internet to both practitioners and users of the service is also seen as driving forward a clinical effectiveness agenda (see Chapter 4).

Increasingly, technology is able to provide either reminders or support in reaching decisions when clinical care is being considered. For example, if you have not been to your general practitioner for some time and you are over a certain age, then he or she will be reminded to offer you a health status check. Women may be routinely invited for cervical screening. Some systems have gone even further. For example, Neural Networks, a type of computer program, can be used to support the diagnosis and treatment of patients with cardiac problems. In this example the computer program examines a wide range of data from patients who have had a confirmed diagnosis of myocardial infarction and is able to identify certain patterns in the data. Links are then formed by the program to represent these patterns, just like the brain establishes a neural network to store information. By entering new data from an undiagnosed case, the program is able to confirm or reject the possibility of the new case also having a myocardial infarct. The decision is still left to the clinician but the machine offers 'advice' based upon up-to-date information on clinically effective care.

Improving quality

A number of approaches have been taken to the improvement of health services. Some are discussed in more detail elsewhere in this book, for example clinical audit (see Chapter 7). Clinical guidelines, protocols and patient care pathways are all playing their part in advancing clinically effective care (Shamian, 1997). These guidelines and pathways are designed by drawing upon the evidential base. This is an area that is likely to expand considerably as a result of the publication of the most recent NHS White Paper (Scottish Office Department of Health, 1997). The introduction of the concept of clinical governance, a renewed focus on quality of care and patient outcome, alongside the desire to deliver seamless services across organisational boundaries, is likely to provide a powerful lever for advancing the clinical effectiveness agenda.

Clinical governance in particular is likely to provide great impetus in driving forward evidence-based care. Although at an early stage of development, it is likely that healthcare providers will be required to give as much attention to the quality of their service as they have done in the past to the financial bottom line. Information on the quality of care will be widely available and so the public will have the opportunity to compare and contrast performance across hospitals. Perhaps, for the first time, the public will have access to information on the effectiveness of treatments. The implication for securing rapid progress, in ensuring that clinically effective care is consistently available, has never been so great.

Overview of levers for clinical effectiveness

The clinical effectiveness agenda is not new: it builds on existing work and is congruent with the underpinning values of professional practice. There are many opportunities and drivers for bringing about clinically effective services. Ultimately, clinical effectiveness is about achieving improved outcomes of care. Figure 5.2 attempts to summarise in graphic terms the material presented in the previous paragraphs in the form of a diagram which illustrates how the various levers of clinical effectiveness may contribute to the ultimate objective of improved clinically effective care.

By clearly identifying the levers for change, nurses in clinical, managerial and educational roles are better placed to understand how the clinical effectiveness agenda can best be progressed within their own sphere of influence. This may entail individual, team or multiprofessional action. It may require fostering the development of alliances across care settings, between organisations, or with patients and public. A multitude of opportunities is available, not least those associated with a revitalised drive to ensure that clinical service quality rather than market competition announced in the White Paper *Designed to Care* (Scottish Office Department of Health, 1997) comes to the fore.

PATHWAYS, GUIDELINES AND PROTOCOLS

Like efficiency, effectiveness and efficacy, a degree of confusion exists regarding the difference between the terms pathways, guidelines and protocols. To a certain extent, pathways, guidelines and protocols are all one and the same thing. They all map a treatment approach for a particular condition or type of client. For some, however, the word 'protocol' is

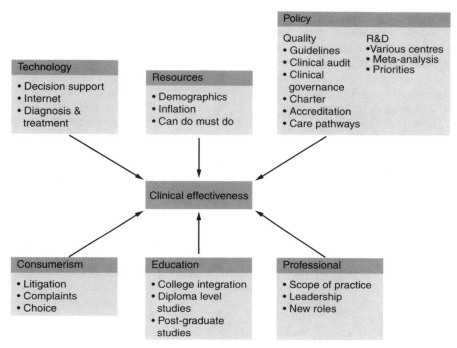

Figure 5.2 Levers to bring about clinically effective care.

unacceptable because of the inferred and actual prescriptive nature. Indeed, the term has a specific legal meaning. In lay terms, a protocol is the prescriptive process to be followed in delivering care for a specific problem or disease. The scope to deviate from the protocol is limited, thereby curtailing the opportunity for the practitioner to exercise judgement. Hence the use of the term 'guideline' and 'care pathway' has been more widely accepted.

GUIDELINES

A wide range of organisations and professional groups targeting particularly diverse topics have produced guidelines. National groups such as the Clinical Outcomes Group (COG) have been proactive in encouraging the development of a number of guidelines, for example the treatment of various forms of cancer.

Clinical guidelines have a history of providing a mechanism for promoting evidence-based practice and a clear avenue for pursuing systematic audit. This is achieved as a result of the guideline offering a written record of the 'state of the science' relating to a particular disease or condition treatment. The guideline acts as an instrument of communication between the scientific community, which produces and synthesises the research-based knowledge, and the practitioners and patients who use and take advantage of the best known treatment modalities.

Despite the value of research-based knowledge there is a long history of the delayed uptake and application of such findings in practice. For example, the work of James Lancaster in 1601 demonstrated the effectiveness of lemon juice in preventing scurvy. The experiment was then repeated almost 150 years later by James Lind, yet it took until the nineteenth century for the British Navy to implement the findings in the prophylactic treatment of the condition.

Many authors have observed that a range of factors can influence the successful uptake of guidelines. In particular, the process followed in the development, dissemination and implementation of the guideline is seen as critical (Haynes *et al.*, 1984; Grimshaw and Russell, 1993a,b, 1994; Haines and Jones, 1994). Grinshaw and Russell (1994) have produced a particularly elegant synopsis of the relative probability of a guidelines uptake, which is summarised in Table 5.1. This table shows that the greater the local ownership of the development process, the more specific the educational intervention for dissemination, and the more patient specific the implementation trigger the more effective the guideline uptake is likely to be.

The advantages and disadvantages of guidelines are similar to those for care pathways; rather than offer unnecessary repetition, the material detailed below should be seen as being equally applicable to guidelines.

Table 5.1 Factors influencing the effectiveness of guidelines (adapted from Grinshaw and Russell, 1994, Achieving health gain through clinical guidelines I. Quality in Health Care, 2, 243–248 with permission from the BMJ Publishing Group)

Relative probability of being effective	Development strategy	Dissemination strategy	Implementation strategy
High	Internal group	Specific educational intervention	Patient-specific reminder at time of consultation or treatment
Above average	Intermediate group	Continuing professional development	Patient-specific feedback
Below average	Local external group	Mailing to targeted groups	General feedback
Low	National external group	Publication in professional journal	General reminder of guideline

CARE PATHWAYS

Care pathways provide a concrete example of how clinically effective care (i.e. patient focused) can be delivered. The approach seeks to describe the services, interventions and expected outcomes that a patient might expect to receive and achieve during treatment for a specific condition.

Benefits of care pathways

Initially much of the development work on guidelines and care pathways focused on a unidisciplinary approach but, because ultimately and ideally care pathways should be patient focused, it was soon recognised that the contributions of an individual profession can deal with only part of patients' needs. Care pathways encourage a holistic analysis of the total needs of the individual, and accordingly care pathways can offer an opportunity for increased multidisciplinary collaboration. Each discipline has a specific contribution to make and, by mapping these carefully, greater understanding and collaboration between disciplines can be achieved.

Similarly, a care pathway does not acknowledge organisational boundaries. It seeks to describe a seamless pathway of care. Accordingly, the contributions, irrespective of organisational source, can be clearly described. By articulating these inputs those involved in the care process, and indeed the individual client, can bring increased pressure to bear, further ensuring that a seamless package of effective care is delivered.

Because the expected outcomes, frequently specified at different stages of the care pathway, are clearly described any deviation or failure to achieve these outcomes or interim goals is quickly identified. Deviations from the expected recovery path therefore provide an early warning so as to trigger any necessary remedial action or at least initiate further assessment and review.

Clear specification of the expected recovery or treatment path that has been optimised by consideration of the research base can result in reduced variations in treatment. The expected interventions and sequence of events are clearly documented; therefore clinicians need to consider carefully before deviating from this path. Variations resultant from individual clinician preferences can therefore be removed unless there is a sound rationale based on unique patient needs.

Inherent in the application of a care pathway approach is a close involvement of the patient or client. By clearly specifying the expected treatment and/or recovery path, patients themselves can play an active part in ensuring optimum treatment regimens are delivered. Patients are far more aware of what is expected and required of professionals as well as the contribution that they themselves can offer. Informed choice and patient partnership becomes a reality. This is, however, an area that still provides significant scope for further development. For example, early editions of the effectiveness bulletin (University of Bristol, 1996; Centre For Reviews and Dissemination, 1997), which sought to describe the state of the clinical treatment science in a number of areas, neglected to provide user-friendly patient information. The responsibility for enacting the scientific base was therefore left solely with professionals. Indeed, only those professionals who had some familiarity with sophisticated meta-analytical techniques may have had the confidence to apply the evidence. Internationally, the Agency for Health Care Policy Research (AHCPR) has taken a slightly wider view. In addition to providing robust meta-analytical publications (AHCPR, 1995, 1996), the AHCPR has also produced more succinct briefing and decision-support materials for hands-on clinicians as well as a parallel document designed to empower patients. By taking this approach, clinicians and patients come jointly to the decision-making process as equal partners. Thankfully, recent editions of the British effectiveness bulletin, such as the publication on benign prostatic enlargement, have started to provide information for clients as well as clinicians.

Although care pathways clearly describe the process of care and indeed those that contribute to its delivery, the system does offer the real opportunity to enact the outcomes-driven approach. Specific goals are stated explicitly. Accordingly, audit against clinical outcome and care delivery process can take place. Furthermore, such audit offers the opportunity for a truly multidisciplinary patient-centred and outcomes-driven approach.

It may well be the case that, on occasion, specific interventions are unable to be offered as the resources may not be available. If this is the case, the care pathway, which monitors deviations from the norm, acts as a powerful tool to identify and quantify any unmet need and resource deficits. This evidence can then be used to realign the resource allocation in a way that was previously dependent on anecdote and a degree of adhocracy.

As well as offering all the previous benefits, care pathways offer the opportunity to deliver the most effective and efficient care. By examining the research evidence closely, pathways can be designed that are underpinned by robust synthesised research results. Indeed, the very process of describing a care pathway can in itself highlight gaps in the evidential base. Simply by asking questions such as 'Why do we do it this way?' and simultaneously turning to the literature, priorities for further research can often be identified.

Drawbacks of care pathways

Care pathways, however, should not be seen as nirvana. They do have their disadvantages as well as the positive points described above.

Clinicians are often uncomfortable with the constraints that a care pathway can bring. A care pathways does not remove the opportunity for clinicians to implement their own preferred treatment regimen, but it certainly does require them to describe and document the rationale for deviating from the agreed optimal care path. There may well be some reasons for doing so: not all patients are the same. For example, co-morbidity or the client's previous clinical history may offer a sound reason for deviation. Another reason for deviation might be the lack of particular resources specified within the care pathway – insufficient staff or the non-availability of a piece of equipment.

Much of the development work relating to care pathways has taken place in the United States. A major driver for the introduction has been the need to control costs. By clearly specifying the care pathway and the associated interventions and diagnostic procedures, unnecessary investigation and/or treatment can be avoided. After all, some investigations do carry with them a significant risk. Despite this fact many clinicians see the pathway as placing a restriction on their freedom to carry out investigations.

Care must be taken to balance the benefits of collecting data and recording progress along the care pathway against the effort and time required to make such recordings, although most advocates of this approach argue that since only deviations need to be recorded time can be saved. However, the analysis of deviations may consume disproportionate resources if complex cases are being treated.

The development of a clinically effective and efficient care pathway does require that an evidential base exist. This is not always the case. Accordingly, expert opinion may need to be sought. Where there is lack of robust evidence, much heated debate can arise.

Developing care pathways

Care pathway development is quite common within UK hospital settings and has often been driven by nursing staff in the first instance. This impetus has came about as a natural extension to the examination and development of evidence-based policies and procedures, often alongside a desire to implement the findings of clinical audit studies. While the detail of the care path and the associated documentation may differ, the process followed in the development of the pathway is relatively consistent.

First, a topic is selected for care pathway development. This topic may be identified for a range of reasons. Often the pathway will cover a high-volume procedure, treatment or clinical problem that is of interest to the clinical team. For example, hip or knee joint replacement, cataract surgery or management of chest pain pathways have commonly been identified as suitable candidates. Usually, there will be some underlying desire to improve the quality of the service being offered so that wide-ranging variations in outcome can be resolved. In addition, and as a result of the introduction of the internal market (Department of Health, 1989), financial reasons may also play a role in topic selection, that is, when variations in treatment regimen may impact on cost for no apparent benefit on outcome.

Second, having identified a topic, the current process or processes are documented, compared and contrasted. What is done? When is it done? Who does it and why? All these questions need to be asked so that a comprehensive picture of current practice can be identified. Having mapped current practice, further questions relating to how the various processes contribute to achieving the final treatment objective must be addressed. Collectively this stage in the process will offer insights into how the existing treatment regimen may be simplified and standardised in such a way as to achieve optimal outcome.

Third, armed with the existing map of care, this can then be compared with published research and subjected to expert views on the topic under consideration. An optimal sequence and timing of diagnostic procedures and treatment interventions can then be developed which minimises delays and resource use whilst maximising quality of care. In short, the care path can be developed. Associated with the path's development is the need at this stage to specify clearly the measures that will be used to assess compliance, timeliness and outcome, as well as the tools needed to gather this information. Care must be taken to ensure that this data collection process adds value rather than an additional burden to those delivering the care. In short, the data should have a clinical use from which management information can be derived.

Fourth, the care pathway then needs to be implemented. This phase of the process must not be neglected. Changing clinical behaviour, as well as possibly learning new skills and knowledge, should not be left to chance. An implementation plan with due regard to the necessary education and training consequences is an essential step.

Fifth, the impact of the introduction of the care pathway should be assessed from a variety of perspectives. Has it reduced unjustified variance in the treatment regimens? Has the quality of care improved and have the predicted changes in outcome transpired? From a managerial stance, has there been more cost-effective use of resources? Such questions need to be asked if the next stage is to be completed. Failure to evaluate the impact of the implementation may result in only partial implementation, regression to former practice or, indeed, unforseen consequences in the changes.

Finally, having evaluated the impact of the introduction of the initial care pathway design, further refinements can be made if necessary. Figure 5.3 seeks to summarise the six-stage process. The process described does not attempt to specify who should be involved in the care pathway design,

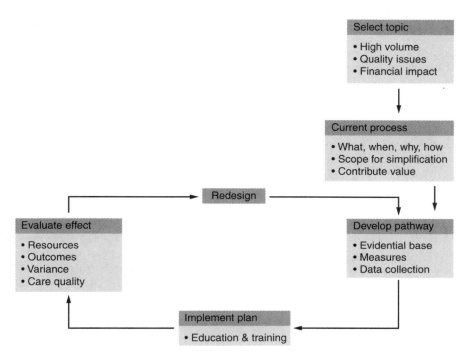

Figure 5.3 Care pathway development.

as this will vary dependent on the topic and scope of the issue to be addressed. However, it is important to note that if you expect people to change their practice for one that purports to be more clinically effective, then the points made in relation to ownership in the above section on guideline development must be considered.

HEALTH GAIN THROUGH CLINICAL EFFECTIVENESS: THE ROLE OF PURCHASING

The 1990 NHS reforms (Department of Health, 1989) introduced the concept of commissioner–provider separation: those who are tasked with assessing the population health needs and buying care for the public are separated from those who offer and deliver the treatment. Despite the recent intention to abandon a market-based approach (Scottish Office Department of Health, 1997) to healthcare, the separation between commissioner and provider continues – all-be-it now in a spirit of partnership. So, while providers must strive to ensure that the care they offer is clinically effective, what is the role of commissioners in progressing this agenda?

Gathering the evidence

Commissioners have to be in a position to understand the implications of advances in medical technology and clinical practice (Littlejohns *et al.*, 1996). New technologies (in the form of drug therapies, surgical procedures, diagnostic equipment, developments in nursing and other techniques) are constantly being developed, and will inevitably create demands on health boards or authorities and the Primary Care Purchasing Cooperative's resources.

Commissioners and providers alike are often critical of the robustness of the evidence available to them. They point to the inadequacies of the research studies that proffer results based on small or unrepresentative samples. Similarly, poorly designed studies or those that do not meet the gold standard of randomised controlled trials can often legitimately present barriers to progress. However, with the changes to the focus of government-funded research, both commissioners and providers can inform the research and development agenda so as to target research funding and effort towards filling gaps in the evidential base. In particular, commissioners might legitimately call for studies that:

- focus upon cost-effectiveness comparisons within disease or client groups so as to assess the effectiveness of different treatment regimens
- develop standardised measures of effectiveness which can then be used routinely to inform the assessment of service performance.

In short, commissioners should be influencing research investment so as to ensure the necessary evidence is available to inform health strategy and purchasing decisions.

Clinically effective systems

Commissioners are in a position to facilitate the development of clinically effective care pathways across organisational boundaries. While professionals are able to develop pathways that are uniprofessional with relative ease, there needs to be wider provider organisational support if multidisciplinary cooperation and agreement is to be reached. If, however, the pathway is to cross organisational boundaries, for example covering the process of care from primary care referral to hospital discharge, then commissioners may need to act as a broker.

As commissioners of care and armed with a sound needs assessment, health boards or authorities and Primary Care Purchasing Cooperatives are in an ideal position to identify gaps and ensure that continuity and consistency of care is facilitated across organisational boundaries. This may entail ensuring that there are incentives for providers to pursue clinically effective systems of care rather than clinically effective elements of care.

The new partnership ways of working, and in particular the synergy between strategic intent described in the Health Improvement Programmes of health boards or authorities and the Trust Implementation Plans, provide an ideal vehicle for such discussion.

Delivering the agenda

To progress the clinical effectiveness agenda from a purchasing perspective there is a need to harness substantial analytical skills, comprising economic, statistical, research, clinical and information analysis skills which are all central to developing an evidence-based approach to commissioning decisions. Some of these resources may be internal to the purchasing organisation, whereas others may be drawn from local providers, acknowledged national experts or educational establishments.

Most commissioners, either explicitly or implicitly via their strategic planning documents such as health improvement programmes, identify the priorities for advancing clinically effective interventions. They frequently specify how, for example, their work in this area can link with that of primary care cooperatives.

Increasingly commissioners are drawing upon a national and international network of resource centres which collate and disseminate information on the various approaches to clinical effectiveness and the associated audit and research and development agendas (see Appendix 1).

Some health boards or authorities have sought to stimulate interest and support developments in the advancement of clinically effective care by sponsoring training programmes or providing earmarked sums of money to bring about change. As well as local provision and formal academic programmes of training, with the advent of new technology some education and training resources are available via the Internet (Table 5.2). Collectively, these approaches help to increase the capacity of both commissioners and providers to engage with a challenging agenda for change.

FUTURE DIRECTIONS FOR CLINICAL EFFECTIVENESS

Over the past several years there has been an increasing emphasis on pursuing and achieving clinically effective care. Resource pressures will undoubtedly continue, and clinicians and mangers alike will be tasked to ensure that the significant health budget is spent wisely. As more and more members of the public gain access to information on what is and is not effective, further pressures will be brought to bear so as to ensure that the most clinically effective treatments are not only offered but delivered. As a result of concepts such as clinical governance introduced in the recent White Paper, policy from government will continue to drive forward

Table 5.2 Iternet Sources of Information on Clinical Effectiveness & Evidence Based Practice	
SOURCE	**DESCRIPTION**
http://www..shef.ac.uk/uni/ academic/r-z/scharr/ir/nett.htm	A valuable resource that gives a list of web site and internet addresses on various aspects of evidence based practice and clinical effectiveness.
http://www.jr2.ox.ac.uk:80/bandolier	A monthly journal published by Oxford and Anglia NHS Executive Regional Office. It covers in a focused manner evidence on the effectiveness of various interventions as well as coverage of methodological issues.
http:/hiru.mcmaster.ca/cochrane. handbook/default.htm	This provides access to a rich source of information on a wide range of material relating to evidence based practice. This covers basic aims of the organisation and ways of establishing review groups right through to practical guidance on establishing registers of review material.
http:/www.ihs.ox.ac.uk/casp/ home_page.html	Provides access to a series of work-shops on critical appraisal skills.
http://www.med.ualberta.ca/ebm/	Gives helpful advice, checklists and methodogical guidance on how to go about conducting a critical review.
http://www.epi.bris.ac.uk/rd/ publicat/ebpurch/index.htm	A bimonthly publication produced by South and West NHS Executive Regional Office targeted towards the needs of commissioners.

further changes. All these factors are likely to result in further evolutionary changes to the way clinical effectiveness is perceived, pursued and delivered.

Box 5.1 highlights some points to discuss in your organisation to ascertain and implement clinically effective care.

Multiprofessional approaches

While many initial developments in the field of clinical effectiveness tended to focus on uniprofessional interventions, more and more attention will in

Box 5.1 Points for discussion

◆ Conduct a PEST (political, economic, social and technological) analysis of the factors that influence your practice

◆ Discuss with colleagues on your ward or clinical service the extent to which clinically effective care is being used

◆ Consider how you might, along with colleagues, identify a topic or area of practice that would be seen as a priority for the implementation of clinically effective care

◆ Reflect upon the levers identified as driving forward clinical effectiveness and assess how you might harness these in bringing about change in your own clinical area

◆ Identify how you might influence the commissioners of care so as to support your efforts in introducing clinically effective care

the coming years be given to multiprofessional collaboration. This will be in response to a patient- rather than profession-focused approach. This will further challenge role boundaries and may require professionals to ask some difficult questions regarding who can deliver the most effective care.

Whole systems approaches

Closely related to the multiprofessional approach is the wider agenda of total systems thinking. Rather than looking at brief episodes of treatment that examine short-term success, increasingly the clinical effectiveness agenda will need to consider the longer-term impact of treatment regimens. This is compatible with the ongoing emphasis on health rather than illness stimulated by the new Green Paper (Scottish Office Department of Health, 1998). Clinical effectiveness across the continuum of care will need to be considered: from primary to secondary and back to primary care.

In addition, the government's recognition that the determinants of health extend way beyond the NHS will also lead to greater cross-organisational initiatives. This is likely to shift the emphasis from clinical effectiveness to health effectiveness. A retrospective example of such an approach arises from looking at effective strategies for dealing with road traffic injury. The introduction of seat belts did more for dealing with flail segment injury than could have been achieved if treatment alone had been considered. In this case the number of such injuries fell dramatically. In short, the further development of the clinical effectiveness agenda will start to encompass aspects of prevention.

At various points in this chapter the concept of 'clinical governance' has been mentioned; although recently introduced in the White Paper *Designed to Care* (Scottish Office Department of Health, 1997), its potential to act as a major driver for clinically effective care should not be underestimated. This concept may provide a major impetus to the further development of the clinical effectiveness agenda as quality, risk and the tapestry of approaches that make up service improvement are all brought together, so that public accountability and scrutiny for value for money rather than cost move to the centre stage. Nurses have traditionally often managed to capture the quality ground, and may have a head start in exploiting this opportunity.

Education and training demands

Clinical effectiveness is still relatively new, and wide-scale integration of the topic into pre and post qualification curricula has, in some programmes, still to take place. It is not simply an additional topic to be taught but a change in the mindset of programme developers that is required. Clinical effectiveness needs to be woven through the very fabric of the programme as well as having specific skills, knowledge and attitude singled out for attention.

As these changes work through the system, nurses as well as other health professionals will need to have far greater access to literature on the effectiveness of the various treatments, interventions and processes. The increased availability of Internet access will help, but sound links with libraries and the expertise that subject specialist librarians offer must not be neglected. Failure to plan for such requirements may delay the everyday implementation of clinically effective care, leading to a patchwork and inconsistent uptake. This may lead to inequities of service.

Public information services

If the public is to make informed choices, to be true partners in the planning of their care and take positive steps towards healthy lifestyles, information must be readily available and easily understood. *Working for Patients* (Department of Health, 1989) coined the phrase that commissioners should be 'champions of the people', yet progress on this agenda has been slow. The information available via the Patients' Charter (Department of Health, 1991) initiative has been severely criticised (Benton, 1993) as not meeting the real needs of the public and also being methodologically flawed. It certainly does not provide the sorts of information that would enable people to judge what is clinically effective care.

While the Agency for Health Care Policy and Research in the USA has from the outset produced patient information on clinically effective interventions as a companion to sophisticated meta-analysis and brief clinician summaries of effectiveness research studies, the UK lags behind. Such information can empower the public, thereby enabling them to ask the 'right' questions of clinicians who offer a treatment. Perhaps this is a development that health commissioners, either individually or better still collectively, might usefully pursue.

As commissioners seek to find new more cost-effective ways of offering services, opportunities might arise that will enable clinically and cost effective care to be introduced from the outset. For example, the nurse telephone helplines announced by government in the recent White Paper that will, in effect, be a pathway-driven approach to care must be seized upon as an opportunity to base advice on the most up-to-data and robust evidence available. Commissioners must not only demand such a stance but also ensure that lessons are more widely learned and applied when other new opportunities such as the functioning of primary care cooperatives is being considered.

CONCLUSION

Clinical effectiveness is here to stay and will continue to evolve into the next millennium. Many potential levers exist for bringing about the reality of consistently available clinically effective care. Healthcare providers and commissioners both have roles to play, as does the general public. The government has signalled its intention to refocus attention on the quality of healthcare services. Professionals therefore have a duty and responsibility to ensure that clinical effectiveness plays its part in pursuing a high-quality cost-effective nationally funded health service.

REFERENCES

Agency for Health Care Policy Research (1995). Patient involvement enhances care for prostate disease. *AHCPR News and Notes*, September 11–12, **187**.
Agency for Health Care Policy Research (1996). *Helping People with Incontinence: Urinary Incontinence, Caregiver Guide*. Washington, DC: Agency for Health Care Policy Research.
Benton, D. (1993). Never mind the quality. *Nursing Standard*, 7(40), 50–51.
Burchfield, R.W. (ed.) (1996). *Fowler's Modern English Usage*. Oxford: Oxford University Press.
Centre for Reviews and Dissemination (1997). Obesity prevention and treatment. *Effective Health Care Bulletin*, **3**, 2.
Department of Health (1989). *Working for Patients*. Cmnd 555. London: HMSO.
Department of Health (1991). *The Patients' Charter*. London: HMSO.
Department of Health (1995). *Improving the Effectiveness of Clinical Services*, Executive Letter EL(95)105. Leeds: NHS Executive.
Department of Health (1996a). *Promoting Clinical Effectiveness: A Framework for Action in and Through the NHS*. Leeds: NHS Executive.
Department of Health (1996b). *Clinical Effectiveness: Reference Pack*, Executive Letter EL(96)110. Leeds: NHS Executive.
Department of Health (1996c). *Complaints: Listening, Acting, Implementing*. London: HMSO.
Department of Health (1997). *NHS Priorities and Planning Guidance 1998/99*, Executive Letter EL(97)39. Leeds: NHS Executive.

Grimshaw, J.M. & Russell, I.T. (1993a). Effect of clinical guidelines on medical practice: a systematic review of rigorous evaluations. *Lancet*, **342**, 1317–1322.

Grimshaw, J.M. & Russell, I.T. (1993b). Achieving health gain through clinical guidelines II – ensuring guidelines change clinical practice. *Quality in Health Care*, **3**, 45–51.

Grimshaw, J.M. & Russell, I.T. (1994). Achieving health gain through clinical guidelines I – developing scientifically valid guidelines. *Quality in Health Care*, **2**, 243–248.

Haines, A. & Jones, R. (1994). Implementing the findings of research. *British Medical Journal*, **308**, 1488–1492.

Haynes, R.B. Roms, D.A. McKibbon, A. & Tugwell, P. (1984). A critical appraisal of the efficacy of continuing medical education. *Journal of the American Medical Association*, **251**, 61–64.

Littlejohns, P. Dumelow, C. & Griffith, S. (1996). Knowledge based commissioning: can a national clinical effectiveness policy be compatible with seeking local professional advice? *Journal of Health Service Research and Policy*, **1**, 28–34.

Scottish Office Department of Health (1997). *Designed to Care: Renewing the National Health Service in Scotland*, Cmnd 3811. Edinburgh: The Stationery Office.

Scottish Office Department of Health (1998). *Working Together for a Healthier Scotland*, Cmnd 3584. Edinburgh: The Stationery Office.

Shamian, J. (1997). How nursing contributes towards quality and cost-effective health care. *International Nursing Review*, **44**, 79–84, 90.

University of Bristol (1996). Total hip replacement. *Effective Health Care Bulletin*, **2**, 7.

6 Development of practice

Lesley Joyce

KEY ISSUES

◆ Definition of practice development

◆ Examination of the contextual siting for the development of practice

◆ Interface between academic and practice settings

◆ Evidence-based approach to the development of practice

◆ Models for developing evidence-based practice

◆ Strategies to be employed in developing evidence-based practice

INTRODUCTION

Development of practice is a much talked about concept but is often ill defined and misunderstood by managers and practitioners alike. Development of practice is about implementing initiatives that promote change or maintain good practice in order to enhance care, and as such should be an essential component in care delivery in any setting.

Practice and professional development are two different concepts, yet in the literature and within job titles they are often used interchangeably. Professional development is concerned with individual practitioners' knowledge, skills and values, and their career development, whereas practice development is concerned with examining and evaluating care delivery in order to improve quality and efficiency. The two are, of course, inextricably linked. If individuals do not consider their own professional development, it is unlikely that they will be effective in the area of practice development. Individuals' skills and knowledge are used in the development of practice. By engaging in practice developments individuals will enhance their professional development.

A definition of practice development is offered by the Royal College of Nursing (1996, p. 4), which describes it as 'a participative client-centred process which integrates research and practice using a range of facilitative methods'. This definition suggests that a major element of development of practice is that of improving quality of care. Development of practice is a complex process in which education, evaluation and research activities should be integrated in order to improve the quality of care delivered. It is not an isolated process rooted in the practice arena, as it aims to bring about clinical innovation and change in light of research evidence and health policy changes (Antrobus and Brown, 1997). Walsh (1995) also supports this view, that the development of practice has a wider role within National Health Service (NHS) development.

Development of practice should be a response to client needs but is also a response to the political context. The changes implemented in the NHS as a response to the 1991 White Paper *Working for Patients* (Department of Health, 1989) produced the superimposition of an internal market. The most influential of these changes was the separation of the purchasing of healthcare from its provision. This has produced the situation whereby purchasers are able to use the 'market' and seek out the most efficient cost-effective care provision. A demand-driven service has been created. This has introduced a culture within care provision where practitioners must understand and more importantly become involved in providing research-based evidence of the effectiveness of practice (Marchment and Hoffmeyer, 1993). In reality practitioners may not feel comfortable engaging within the commissioning process, and it may not be appropriate for them to become involved at that level. Practitioners can, though, be very influential in providing the information regarding clinical practices and the evidence to support those practices, which is needed to inform the commissioning process. Walsh (1995) suggests that academic staff can act as 'brokers' within the commissioning process by translating practice evidence into language that is understood within the commissioning agenda. Such a liaison can help practitioners to learn the political language and so gain a voice within the political debate.

A consequence of the recent change in government appears to be that there will be changes to the internal market system over the coming years. Yet it will remain a priority within practice that practitioners can provide the evidence to support their practices and continue to develop all elements of care delivery. In all clinical environments practitioners are having to cope with increased workloads and in many instances increased client dependency. Such working practices mean that practitioners must consider development of practice as of paramount importance. Development of practice should not be viewed as a short-term strategy for overcoming immediate problems. A long-term, planned and organised approach should be adopted so that initiatives that are developed will survive and continue to develop.

DEVELOPING A CULTURE TO SUPPORT PRACTICE DEVELOPMENT

In order to support the development of practice, the clinical environment should be one in which ideas, innovations and research are valued. It is all too easy to become so involved in day to day caring that evidence-based practice is neglected. Practitioners can become so busy caring for patients that they have no time for research (Wright and Dolan, 1991), especially if there is not a culture to support evidence-based practice. Walsh (1997) identifies the clinical environment as one of the major barriers to implementing research.

There may be conflict surrounding the implementation of evidence-based practice, and Macguire (1990) suggests that there may be resistance to utilising research because of the differing goals held by the power groups in large organisations. The main function of implementing evidence-based practice should be to improve care for the clients. As practitioners are often most involved in care delivery they should feel empowered to implement evidence-based practice. They need to have real power in order to implement change, especially as evidence-based practice lays the accountability with individual practitioners. Accountability means that practitioners will be able to give an explanation of and justification for their actions (Walsh, 1997). This accountability does not have to rest upon changing major areas of practice but may be at the level of the practitioner being able to decide which evidence is relevant. To do this, practitioners will require the skills to evaluate evidence. Once confident in these skills, practitioners can then be encouraged and supported to gain the skills required to undertake the change process needed to implement evidence-based practice.

Often this progression is overlooked and practitioners are expected to develop practice with no education or support. Development of practice requires the practitioner to possess many skills. You need to acquire and develop skills in negotiating, selling, cooperation and, importantly, risk taking.

Individual practitioners are often enthusiastic regarding development of practice yet will require continued support to retain their motivation. Part of this support can be gained through links with higher education organisations. If there is a culture of mutual support and collaboration built between higher education and service deliverers, then the implementation of evidence-based practice can be enhanced. Time will be required to develop such relationships with a real commitment from both areas. The setting up of joint projects can be a way to involve both organisations. It is important that the evidence being sought is not just for academic credibility but that the project is undertaken with the aim of informing and developing practice. As such, it is an advantage when practice informs and directs the project. As practitioners it is important that you inform the educationalists what are the real issues to be investigated.

Reflection   Try to identify your links with educational organisations. What are the strengths of this relationship and how can they be developed further?

At present the way that most educationalists will be involved in links with service areas is through student support. Often this is not successfully operated and possibly does little to support the development of practice. One way adopted by the writer to enhance the process has been to develop a tripartite approach, involving nursing students, clinical staff and educationalists. Regular meetings are set up where all parties attend to discuss and reflect upon critical incidents that have occurred in practice. This approach has had a very positive effect upon building relationships, as well as enhancing care delivery. There is the opportunity for the educationalist to link theory to real practice issues and for students and clinical staff to examine practice. The clinicians are challenged to support their decisions and provide a rationale for actions. The students benefit from the presence of a member of the clinical staff and all meetings take place within the clinical area. This is a simple strategy but as such educationalists are seen to be removed from their ivory towers. These meetings can be challenging for all present and it is important that the clinical member and educationalist are both suitably experienced to support the students and each other, in what can potentially be very emotional and threatening experiences.

In a culture where cost-cutting exercises are the norm and resources are limited, funding to support the development of research-based practice may not be top of the agenda. There may therefore be a need for practitioners to be creative in obtaining funding and time to support the development of evidence-based practice. There are many agencies offering support and funding to which practitioners can turn, as outlined in a previous chapter. The White Paper *The New NHS: Modern, Dependable* (Department of Health, 1997) clearly sets an agenda of raising care standards and sets out that each Trust will have a legal responsibility for quality (Jay, 1997). The new reforms will focus on quality, accountability and clinical effectiveness. The government is supporting these aims by setting up two new bodies: the National Institute for Clinical Excellence and a new Commission for Health Improvement. Both bodies will offer support in the development of practice.

THE EVIDENCE-BASED APPROACH TO THE DEVELOPMENT OF PRACTICE

Within the process of practice development there is a need to identify the relevance of evidence-based practice to the practitioner's everyday role and function. Rosenberg and Donald (1995) suggest that there are many advantages to practising evidence-based medicine, not only for the clients but also for individual practitioners and multidisciplinary teams. By using evidence-based practice, individual practitioners can improve their knowledge base, which in turn gives them the confidence in their clinical decision making. The benefits to care delivery teams is that evidence-based practice can provide a framework within which the team can operate.

A further benefit of utilising evidence-based practice is related to teaching. By using an evidence-based practice approach, new and junior team members can not only learn and develop skills but also they have the opportunity to contribute to team decisions. Newly qualified staff should, by the nature of their education, possess skills in searching for and critically analysing clinical evidence. They should therefore be encouraged to continue to develop their skills and contribute to the team by collecting and critically appraising clinical evidence which can then be used to inform care delivery. The skills possessed by newly qualified staff should be utilised to help more senior staff to develop such skills. Pearcey (1995) researched practitioners' attitudes towards evidence-based practice and found that nurses who had trained recently or who had undergone some form of postregistration education demonstrated more favourable attitudes than established staff who had not undertaken any recent education.

BEST PRACTICE

The Department of Health (1996) defines clinical effectiveness as 'the extent to which specific clinical interventions when deployed for a particular patient or population do what they are intended to do'. Within practice and care delivery there is a need to understand how evidence links with the implementation and monitoring of clinical effectiveness. This is becoming increasingly important as practitioners are constantly being asked to define the effectiveness of their interventions not only by their managers but also by the purchasers of care. Within the existing internal market such proof of effectiveness has to be presented to external purchasers, such as consortia and general practitioners. Perhaps more importantly, practitioners should also be utilising evidenced-based practice to prove the effectiveness of their chosen interventions to the recipients of care. Within the bounds of practice development, utilising evidence-based practice means being able to explain to clients why certain interventions are being used and what their expected outcomes are. Morgan (1997) writes that in order to utilise evidence-based practice practitioners need first to be able to define what it is, what are the different levels of evidence and how to access the various sources of evidence, all of which have been examined in previous chapters.

Evidence in the context of practice development should relate to 'best practice', in other words the best action, process or particular treatment relative to individual clients or groups of clients.

Reflection   How do you as practitioners decide upon what is best practice? Do you adopt routine practices or do you challenge rituals within your practice? Write down one or more specific interventions for which you can identify the evidence base. Where did you obtain this evidence? What process was used to implement any changes needed?

Previous chapters have identified and examined techniques for searching, collecting and critically evaluating the evidence related to effective practice. These are all important stages in the process of implementing an evidence-based approach. In relation to practice development one of the most important stages is utilising the evidence. Many practitioners, as a result of their education, are becoming skilled in collecting and critically appraising the evidence but there appears too often to be a problem when it comes to implementing the evidence in practice. The evidence must be used to inform practitioners' interventions if practice is to be developed. One element of practice development is utilising the most appropriate available evidence as part of the clinical decision-making process.

A problem-solving approach can aid the implementation of the findings. By utilising search and retrieval techniques the evidence to support the identified interventions can be sought and, once collected, the evidence should be appraised critically. If the evidence is found to be reliable, valid and, importantly, appropriate to your clinical situation, then it can be used to support existing interventions or to facilitate the implementation of new interventions.

MODELS FOR DEVELOPING EVIDENCE-BASED PRACTICE

This continual drive for quality and effectiveness within the delivery of care has reinforced the need for evidence-based practice. In a practice context, evidence is often regarded by practitioners as scientific knowledge or research findings. Yet there are within practice many other forms of evidence upon which to develop good practice (see Box 6.1), for example the evidence derived from culture, custom and narratives or that relating to anecdotes from experience. Such evidence often has a strong influence upon the development of practice, most likely through the medium of role

Box 6.1 Summary of models for developing evidence-based practice

Role modelling   Skills are learnt from another practitioner, by watching the practice and actions of that practitioner.

Reflection on action   Practice is examined after it has occurred.

Action learning groups   Groups of practitioners meet to discuss issues and, more importantly, to set action plans to develop practice.

Research awareness groups   Groups are set up to discuss research articles and reports critically and to examine their implications for practice.

modelling. This is often one of the most influential ways in which new practitioners develop their practice.

Schon (1987) recognised the importance of practice-based evidence and suggested that if only a scientific approach is applied to practice the humanness within care delivery can be lost. It is important that as practitioners you do not let scientific findings totally override your own experiences of working with clients. By using the skill of reflecting upon practice, practitioners can utilise their experiences and derive personal theories developed from working with clients. Part of the process of reflection should be to link knowledge and theory to experience. This will help you as a practitioner to identify and justify the source of your knowledge, which has informed your actions and decision making.

By using a systematic process of reflection, practitioners can make sense of their practice and continue to develop practice in a meaningful and constructive manner. Constructive reflection involves analysis and interpretation of practice, which requires the acquisition of complex skills. Practitioners will require help and support to be able to develop such skills. There is a wealth of literature on 'How to Reflect', which can help the practitioner gain such skills. This can be a time-consuming process. If undertaken alone, solitary reflection may be counterproductive; practitioners can be very self-effacing and focus upon negative aspects when reflecting upon their performance. In many circumstances peer group reflection can be more productive. Such an activity requires time and support, and the process needs to be approved within the work environment. A further element that can enhance the peer group reflective process is experienced facilitation. If left to their own devices a reflective peer group can use the time to 'whine and whinge' rather than to examine and explore practice in order to develop care delivery. Facilitation can be offered by an academic link, where a lecturer meets peer groups on a regular basis. This can help bridge the theory–practice gap. The academic support person will need to possess the theoretical base as well as appropriate clinical experience and communication skills in order to facilitate a systematic approach to the reflective process. Such an activity can enhance the development of practice as well as strengthen the academic and clinical link. This activity can provide mutual gain for all concerned if certain ground rules are adhered to.

Points to consider when setting up peer reflection:

- approved time away from clinical area where group are not disturbed
- regular meetings to allow for the formation of relationships
- confidentiality and trust are essential
- facilitation of a creative and challenging environment, not to support the *status quo*
- production of action plans
- support by management for the process.

What have been described are also known as action learning groups.

Reflection   Think about the process that has been described. How would you set up your own action learning group? Who would be involved? Where would the meetings be held? What problems might you encounter and how could you overcome them?

Action learning groups can inform a practice development model, where strategies of change are derived from everyday practice. When such an activity leads to the development of theory, the process can be described as an inductive approach to forming evidence (Kitson *et al.*, 1996). This approach takes account of the practice context and acknowledges the practitioner's interpretations of events. These then become an integral part of the change process. Although such an approach is significant in developing practice, what is often lacking is a systematic approach and, more importantly, formal reporting of the process. As practitioners it is important that you learn to think through your actions and record the process of change. You need to collect evidence to justify your actions and also to identify clearly and objectively the benefits of the change, especially in terms of benefit to clients. A good way of doing this is to involve the clients: they are the best ones to identify the benefits.

The inductive phase can be supplemented by following the process with a deductive phase (Kitson *et al.*, 1996). This involves hypothesis testing, i.e. a testing and evaluation of the changes. This can be carried out in an individual approach, where the practitioner works through the interventions again and tests for the same outcome, or by a peer approach, where a group of practitioners tests out the theory. What should occur in either situation is a formal evaluation; again, recording is crucial to the process.

Another way to help facilitate practice development, in a group situation, is by setting up research awareness groups. A group of practitioners would meet, in this context with a specific intention. The group's aim would be critically to evaluate pieces of written evidence to support their practice. The group membership does not necessarily have to be a peer group: in fact, it may be more appropriate for the group to be multidisciplinary. Before each meeting the group would need to decide upon a topic for discussion and who would be responsible for bringing the evidence to discuss. This may be individuals or small groups of people, who bring evidence for the whole group to examine critically and, most importantly, for the group to discuss the implications of the evidence to practice. The group will possibly benefit from the attendance of an experienced facilitator, at least at the first meetings. Bassett (1992) supports the journal club approach as being of benefit in the development of evidence-based practice.

Reflection   Read each of the models again and decide upon a model that would be appropriate within your clinical setting. How would you implement such a model?

PRACTICE DEVELOPMENT: ADOPTING AN AUDIT APPROACH

Practice development is a dynamic process and requires a constant evaluation in the form of audit. As such, the process should be continuous and practitioners should constantly be examining the effectiveness of their interventions and whole care-delivery approach. There is a danger that practice development can become the in thing to do and, as such, the process takes place purely for the sake of change alone. This can often mean that practitioners feel that they are playing the game of 'catch up', and the purpose of practice development is lost.

The central purpose of practice development is to ensure the best care is delivered in the most appropriate and effective manner. Audit of practice is therefore an integral component of practice development and is discussed in detail in Chapter 7. A consideration of the role audit can play, specifically in relation to practice development, needs to be examined here. Audit is a formal process by which the effectiveness of interventions is tested. By utilising such a process it may be found that existing practice is already best practice and a change is not at present needed. This is perfectly acceptable and is important within practice development. It is important for practitioners not to rest on their laurels but continually to seek out and critically examine new evidence. The evidence identified should then be tested against existing practice, and such practice changed whenever it is found to be no longer appropriate. It should be the responsibility of all practitioners to utilise effective evidence-based practice as soon as it becomes available. This requires a degree of effort on the part of each practitioner to be aware of new evidence as it is released. Practice development is not a one-off process but should be dynamic.

Another way of identifying areas for potential change in practice, often encompassed within the audit process, is via the controversial route of using the monitoring of errors. Meurier, Vincent and Posmar (1997) carried out a study which examined the use of this technique and found that the most common causes of error were lack of knowledge or information, work overload, stressful atmosphere and lack of support from senior staff. It is of course important to identify and correct errors within practice, yet it is the approach used to do this that is crucial. It would appear that it is important to examine the errors in relation to their impact upon the quality of care. This can be achieved by drawing on relevant evidence in relation to why errors occur in certain situations. Often what occurs is a focusing upon the individual who committed the error. In this situation the individual is most likely to become defensive and as a consequence he or she may in the future cover up errors for fear of retribution. It is more important to foster a positive developmental approach and to help facilitate a self-critical approach to practice, supporting and enabling practitioners to be aware and become personally accountable for their own actions. It is more beneficial to create an atmosphere where learning from errors occurs and practitioners learn to utilise relevant evidence upon which to base their decisions. They can become skilled in employing a problem-solving approach and examining relevant evidence to promote positive changes within practice. Reflection upon the situation can be a powerful tool in helping the practitioner to identify why a situation occurred and how to avoid a recurrence.

Reflection   Figures are often collected of errors made and these are used as a basis for changing practice. How do you feel about this approach to changing practice?

Think of a time when you or a colleague made an error. How was the situation handled? Did the incident lead to a defensive or constructive change in practice? How would you have managed the situation?

IMPLEMENTING EVIDENCE-BASED PRACTICE

Errors may occur as a result of the practitioner not having the correct information upon which to make a decision. This can be due to inexperience or lack of support to enable the practitioner to gain the information. It is every practitioner's responsibility to gain access to the relevant evidence upon which to base practice. There is an increasing body of evidence now becoming available, yet a limited amount of this empirical knowledge is being used in practice (Burns and Grove, 1993). So, despite evidence becoming more readily available to all practitioners, practice that is out-dated and at worst dangerous may continue to be implemented.

Reflection   You may think that the last statement sounds harsh. Think about your own practice. Are there practices and/or interventions that are being continued despite you knowing that they are not based upon evidence? List any such practices or interventions. Now, think about why the practice or intervention has not changed.

By examining your list of reasons you will see that what you have identified are the barriers and restrictions to implementing evidence-based practice. What you have identified is also known as the evidence–practice gap. It has been suggested by Taylor (1997) that the evidence-based approach to practice delivery can be a way to integrate theory and practice successfully.

This gap can exist for many reasons, and elements of the failure to bridge the gap can be attributed to both practitioners and researchers.

Practitioners:

- may not make efforts to keep up to date with new evidence
- may be comfortable with traditional or ritual practices
- may lack the resources, especially time, to find the evidence
- may lack confidence to change practice
- may encounter restrictions within the organisation to change practice.

Researchers (evidence providers):

- Evidence may be disseminated poorly or not at all. Often researchers do not write up and publish their research findings, especially students undertaking courses.
- Published material does not target the practitioners in a manner appropriate to their needs.
- The time gap between finding the evidence and publishing the findings is long.
- The language used is not understandable by the reader.
- The report does not address the implications for practice.

Walsh (1997) suggests that more practitioners are becoming aware of the need to base practice upon relevant and appropriate research. Yet difficulties remain in implementing such evidence into practice. From her research, Lacey (1994) found that nurses identified the barriers as lack of time to read research findings and lack of resources. It is very easy to look at the barriers, yet a more fundamental problem may be that for some areas there is little or no evidence available. Practitioners should not become discouraged when they cannot find empirical evidence to support their practice.

In this situation, as a practitioner, there are two choices: to do nothing or to pursue the search for evidence-based practice. By the fact that you are reading this book you are more likely to opt for the second choice. But what do you do? You need to start by examining your practice:

- Identify an area of practice that troubles you. One way to do this might be to think of a practice that can be attributed to custom or ritual.
- By following the advice given in previous chapters, search out the literature relevant to this practice.
- Read and critically evaluate the literature identified.
- Share the information with colleagues.
- Compare your practice with that suggested in the literature.
- Does a change need to be made?
- If so, how will you do this?

You may well be thinking that is an awful lot to do, but once you have worked through the process once it will become easier. Remember that there will be other people who have done this before, so seek their help.

STRATEGIES FOR DEVELOPING 'BEST PRACTICE'

Clinical guidelines

When appropriate evidence has been collected and appraised it can be utilised to support the development of clinical guidelines. National guidelines may already exist for certain areas of practice. Nationally devised guidelines will have collated and used all the existing evidence related to a specific client group of intervention. These guidelines should represent the highest level of evidence. Clinical guidelines at a local level can provide standards of care which are agreed by unidisciplinary or multidisciplinary groups. When evidence based, clinical guidelines can provide expert knowledge in an easily accessible format which can be used by practitioners to inform their interventions. Such guidelines can facilitate the raising of care standards and help practitioners to prove the effectiveness of their interventions. The National Institute for Clinical Excellence will be instrumental in issuing clinical guidelines on relevant evidence of clinical and cost effectiveness.

All practitioners need to be involved in the development of evidence-based guidelines and not allow medicine and doctors to dictate the practice development process. When ready-made guidelines do not exist, practitioners should seek out systematic reviews of evidence relating to a specific area or topic (e.g. Abu-Saad and Hamers, 1997). These provide summaries and overviews of the research available within the specific area. Practitioners should then collate and analyse the available evidence. Once the appropriate evidence has been identified, it must be converted into a useable medium, such as clinical guidelines.

Practice development leaders

Practice development is the most challenging part of achieving the NHS clinical effectiveness agenda according to Walsh (1995), because traditionally no systems have existed for managing the process of clinical change. At present there are no standard applications for implementing practice development.

Many organisations have decided to appoint specific personnel with responsibility for leading practice development in clinical areas. Such individuals carry titles such as practice development officers, clinical specialists or lecturer practitioners. Just as there are many titles, there are also many interpretations of the role. Some individuals carry a managerial responsibility as well as a practice development role; others have no such responsibility and no access to resources such as budgets or human resources. Practice development leaders have to be capable of motivating and educating others as well as leading changes in practice. It is a role for which people should be carefully chosen and prepared. Getting the right person for the job can make the difference between successful or unsuccessful practice development. These roles are often operated within a very complex hierarchy and achieve a variety of successes.

The main problems with such roles appear to be:

• poor access to resources
• poor managerial support
• mixed agendas as a result of working for many agents
• limited time allowed for release of staff to undertake projects
• inadequate training or preparation for the role.

When individuals are employed to lead practice development they are expected to act as agents for change, encouraging evidence-based practice and facilitating the audit process. It is important that such roles do not overshadow individual practitioners, who can have a major role in practice development.

Development units

Many organisations have implemented very successful support for practice development. Perhaps the most well publicised are the nursing and practice development units that have been set up around the country. In 1992 the Department of Health funded the setting up of more than 30 nursing development units across a range of settings. Johnson (1989) described the aim of nursing development units as the development of nurses and of nursing practice. Turner-Shaw and Bosanquet (1993) suggested that the setting up of such units would meet a professionalising agenda, but in practice may mean the development of high-quality care in disparate pockets. Salvage (1989) supported this view in describing the units as limiting and elitist. Indeed, development units do offer the potential for high-quality care, but in reality this best practice is not disseminated beyond the bounds of the units. Secretary of State for Health Frank Dobson (1997) criticised the poor dissemination of best practice and advocated a system whereby examples of good practice must be shared. This is a strategy that should be adopted by all professions. Naish (1997) suggested that, at present, professional jealousy can be a destructive emotion which hinders practice development.

Practice development units share the innovative approach to care delivery but recognise the importance of a multidisciplinary team approach. They aim to develop a culture that is egalitarian, delegates power downwards, and encourages a wide range of staff members to be involved in decision making (Williams and Lowry, 1993).

Dissemination of good practice

An area where there is often a poor dissemination of evidence is from the academic to the practice setting. This occurs not only as a dissonance between academic researchers and practice-based practitioners, but by practitioners themselves. When practitioners undertake courses they often have to undertake a research project as part of the assessment strategy. Often these projects do not link real clinical problems to the academic process. This can be overcome by practitioners thinking clearly about what are the real issues in practice, and academics encouraging practitioners to investigate those real issues. Mulhall (1997, p. 970) argued that this continues to be a problem: 'the discipline-orientated university and the practice-orientated service continue to hold different values and beliefs'.

Even when practitioners do investigate real practice issues they often do not share their findings; nor do they write research articles (Hicks, 1995). Research articles are often written by academics, who are required as part of their role to produce publications. This produces a particular emphasis in the writing which may not be appropriate for practitioners to transfer the findings into the clinical setting. It is important that writing and publishing by practitioners comes to be seen as an important aspect of practice development. Haines and Jones (1994) discuss the cultural divide between researchers, practitioners and educators when reporting upon research, and believe that a way to bridge this divide is to consider research as the common denominator and something that must be shared by all. A common language should be adopted so that all interested parties can understand and interpret the evidence. Closs and Cheater (1994) agree that the way in which research findings are reported often presents a major barrier to implementation. Two strategies for improving the written report are by attending to the content and to the style (Mulhall, 1997). A simple strategy is to ask the question: 'Who am I writing this for?' and therefore to consider what information they require and how they will want to use the information. When practitioners do become involved in research they can become part of this research culture, yet, as Hardy and Mulhall (1994) suggest, for various reasons it is neither desirable nor practical for all practitioners to undertake research. The responsibility for making explicit the evidence, in terms that are understandable by practitioners, often then lies with the researcher and academics.

Networking

So far dissemination has been referred to in terms of the written word. Another strategy is via person-to-person contact (Black, 1992), also defined as networking – the sharing of information and innovations within and without your organisation. Interestingly, although simple, it is a strategy that often does not occur. Researchers and practitioners may become very protective about their innovations and evidence, not wanting to share. This has its origins within professional boundaries but has been strengthened by the competitive element embodied within the internal market philosophy introduced into care delivery. Networking can be a very positive strategy, offering support as well as information. Black (1992) advocates the setting up of networks in order to share experiences, exchange ideas and develop contacts.

Reflection   Spend a few minutes identifying your own networks. How do you communicate with these people? Think about how you can extend your network.

Networking often occurs when people come together because they have a common interest concerning practice development, for example around developing primary nursing. Like-minded people may meet or communicate via the telephone or e-mail system to share information and ideas. Such networking can be very useful if you are in the early stages of developing an innovation. This support can save you time in finding supporting evidence and, perhaps more importantly, can save you the effort of not making similar mistakes.

There are, of course, some barriers towards setting up network systems. These include the philosophy of competition enhanced within the quasi-market environment. This may be a situation that improves as the changes proposed by the Labour government take a hold. Also, poor communication skills can hamper the networking process, either within organisations or by individuals themselves. This may be due to poor skills such as the inability to use information technology or a lack of confidence.

Research summaries

Perhaps we have not yet identified the most fundamental question. How do you as practitioners find the time to read all the evidence in order to inform your practice development? Even if the reports are written in a style appropriate to your needs, it would be impossible to read all of them, even those specifically related to your topic areas. We have already suggested the research awareness group as a way of sharing the evidence. Another technique has been addressed within many professional journals where summaries of reports are presented. By reading these you will be able to identify those most relevant to your practice and then read the full report of fewer articles, so cutting down the time required. You will need to be able to evaluate critically each report you read before considering the usefulness of the evidence in relation to your practice. Just because an article is published does not mean necessarily that the evidence is reliable or valid: you must decide this for yourself. We have experienced the situation where an article was read by a group of practitioners and the evidence used to change clinical practice. The evidence was actually very poor and led to a change in practice where the effectiveness was lower than that of the practice previously implemented. Cooper (1989) stresses the need for practitioners to explore several related studies and to draw overall conclusions rather than relying on only one piece of evidence.

Action research

Action research is a strategy that can offer practitioners the opportunity to identify areas of concern within their own practice and find solutions to overcome problems. It is a strategy that occurs within practice and is carried out by practitioners. Many practitioners do not feel confident to initiate such projects and will require help. This is a further opportunity for educationalists and clinicians to work together. Educationalists who possess research skills must be encouraged to undertake projects based in the practice environment (Kitson *et al.*, 1996).

Walsh (1997) believes that research needs to be done by some, facilitated by others, and implemented by all. Confidence in your own ability to change practice is essential to practice development.

A culture of sharing is also essential: there needs to be involvement and cooperation with all working in the healthcare system. This may not be an easy or quick fix process, as it may mean that professional barriers have to be broken down. By working together on projects, professionals can learn to share and develop evidence that is relevant to all groups. There is a need to develop multidisciplinary evidence-based initiatives and, more importantly, a culture where all individuals are fully cooperative and sharing.

CONCLUSION

In conclusion, this chapter has highlighted the factors essential to the process of practice development (see Box 6.2).

Box 6.2 Factors essential to practice development

Evidence The need to identify relevant and valid evidence is crucial and requires the practitioner to develop a set of skills in order to achieve this. For certain areas evidence may not be available; practitioners should then seriously consider defining their own evidence to support their practice.

Empowerment Practitioners need to be empowered to be involved in decision making. Power and authority need to be devolved. Individuals have to be ready to accept individual accountability.

Creativity Practice development requires a challenging attitude and, at times, risk taking.

Teamwork Practice development can be best achieved within a collaborative framework, where sharing expertise and knowledge are commonplace. This requires shared responsibility and shared leadership.

Resources These are economic and human. Time is one of the most crucial.

Environment There needs to be a supportive culture in which there is an open and honest atmosphere.
There needs to be a consistency of approach to evidence-based practice.

Education All practitioners should have the opportunity to be supported to achieve the skills required to implement evidence-based practice.

Dissemination Communication links to share evidence should occur locally, nationally and internationally.

Reflections   At the end of this chapter it may be useful to pose several questions that all practitioners should ask of themselves:

- What is the evidence that I use to frame my working practice?
- How do I keep up to date with the ever-increasing amount of evidence available?
- Do I reflect upon and evaluate the care that I give?
- How can I work with others to develop practice in our work setting?

REFERENCES

Abu-Saad, H.H. & Hamers, J. (1997). Decision-making and paediatric pain: a review. *Journal of Advanced Nursing*, **26**(5), 946–952.

Antrobus, S. & Brown, S. (1997). The impact of the commissioning agenda upon nursing practice: a proactive approach to influencing health policy. *Journal of Advanced Nursing*, **25**, 309–315.

Bassett, C. (1992). The integration of research in the clinical setting: obstacles and solutions. A review of the literature. *Nursing Practice*, **6**(1), 4–8.

Black, F. (1992). Networking for change. *Nursing Times*, **88**(1), 58–59.

Burns, N. & Grove, S. (1993). *The Practice of Nursing Research: Conduct, Critique and Utilisation*. London: Saunders.

Closs, J. & Cheater, F. (1994). Utilisation of nursing research: culture, interest and support. *Journal of Advanced Nursing*, **19**, 762–773.

Cooper, H.M. (1989). *Integrating Research – A Guide for Literature Reviews*, 2nd edn. Newbury Park: Sage.

Department of Health (1989). *Working for Patients*. London: HMSO.

Department of Health (1996). *Promoting Clinical Effectiveness: A Framework for Action In and Through the National Health Service*. London: HMSO.

Department of Health (1997). *The New NHS: Modern, Dependable*. London: HMSO.

Dobson F. (1997). Spreading the word. *The Times on Sunday*, 19 October.

Haines, A. & Jones, R. (1994). Implementing findings of research. *British Medical Journal*, **308**, 1488–1492.

Hardy, M. & Mulhall, A. (1994). *Nursing Research, Theory and Practice*. London: Chapman Hall.

Hicks, C. (1995). The shortfall in published research: a study of nurses' research and publication activities. *Journal of Advanced Nursing*, **21**, 594–604.

Jay, M. (1997). Guest Editorial: The White Paper recognises that nurses have a critical contribution to make. *Nursing Times*, **93**(51), 3.

Johnson, M. (1989). Challenge of the new. *Health Service Journal*, **99**(5231), 178.

Kitson, A., Ahmed, L., Harvey, G., Seers, K. & Thompson, D. (1996). From research to practice: one organisational model for promoting research-based practice. *Journal of Advanced Nursing*, **23**(3), 430–440.

Lacey, A. (1994). Research utilisation in nursing practice: a pilot study. *Journal of Advanced Nursing*, **19**, 987–997.

Macguire, J. (1990). Putting research findings into practice: research utilisation as an aspect of the management of change. *Journal of Advanced Nursing*, **15**, 614–620.

Marchment, M. & Hoffmeyer, V. (1993). Towards a formalisation of quality in health care contracts. *Health Service Management Research*, Part 4, 4 November, 229–236.

Meurier, C., Vincent, C. & Posmar, D. (1997). Learning from errors in nursing practice. *Journal of Advanced Nursing*, **26**, 111–119.

Morgan, E. (1997). Clinical effectiveness. *Nursing Standard*, **11**(34), 43–50.

Mulhall, A. (1997). Nursing research: our world not theirs? *Journal of Advanced Nursing*, **25**, 969–976.

Naish, J. (1997). A lost opportunity. *Nursing Standard*, **11**(25), 17.

Pearcey, P. (1995). Achieving research based nursing practice. *Journal of Advanced Nursing,* **22**, 33–39.

Rosenberg, W. & Donald, A. (1995). Evidence-based medicine: an approach to clinical problem solving. *British Medical Journal,* **310**, 1122–1126.

Royal College of Nursing (1996). *The RCN Clinical Effectiveness Initiative: A Strategic Framework.* London: RCN.

Salvage J (1989) Building centres of excellence. *Nursing Standard,* **3**(48), 53–56.

Schon, D. (1987). *Educating the Reflective Practitioner.* San Francisco: Jossey Bass.

Taylor, M.C. (1997). What is evidence-based practice? *British Journal of Occupational Therapy,* **60**(11), 470–474.

Turner-Shaw, J. & Bosanquet, N. (1993). *Nursing Development Units: A Way to Develop Nurses and Nursing.* London: Kings Fund.

Walsh, K. (1995). Given in evidence. *Health Service Journal,* **105**, 28–29.

Walsh, M. (1997). How nurses perceive barriers to research implementation. *Nursing Standard,* **11**(29), 34–39.

Williams, C. & Lowry, M. (1993). Practice development units: the next step? *Nursing Standard,* **8**(11), 25–29.

Wright, S. & Dolan, M. (1991). Coming down from the ivory tower. *Professional Nurse,* October, 38–41.

Further reading

Black, M. (1994). *Networking.* London: Kings Fund.

Ersser, S, Tutton, L. & Salvage, J. (1990). A network for change. *Nursing Times,* **86**, 28–29.

Kitson, A. (1997). Developing excellence in nursing practice and care. *Nursing Standard,* **12**(2), 33–37.

Luker, K.A. & Kendrick, M. (1992). An exploratory study of the sources of influence on the clinical decisions of community nurses. *Journal of Advanced Nursing,* **17**, 457–466.

Stocking, B. (1992). Promoting change into critical care. *Quality in Health Care Journal,* 1, 56–60.

Tierney, A. & Taylor, J. (1991). Research in practice: an experiment in researcher–practitioner collaboration. *Journal of Advanced Nursing,* **16**, 506–570.

Watt, G. (1993). Making research make a difference. *Health Bulletin,* **57**, 187–195.

Weir, P. & Kendrick, K. (1994). Setting up networks to improve practice. *Nursing Standard,* **8**(41), 29–33.

Wilson-Barnett, J., Corner, J. & De Carle, B. (1990). Integrating nursing research and practice: the role of the researcher as teacher. *Journal of Advanced Nursing,* **15**, 621–662.

7 Audit

Gayle Garland and Fran Corfield

KEY ISSUES

◆ Stages in the audit process

◆ Benefits of clinical audit

◆ Challenges within the audit process

◆ Accountability and audit

INTRODUCTION

Audit serves the vital function of testing and confirming that clinically effective care is being provided. It is a tool to measure how well you are meeting the standards you have set for clinical care on a day-to-day basis. The analysis of audit findings determines whether praise or improvement is needed (NHS Executive, 1998a). Evaluation of care has always been an integral part of professional practice. The emphasis now is on formalised and comprehensive evaluation: providing evidence to demonstrate that quality care is, or is not, being both attained and maintained (Luthert and Robinson, 1993).

Clinical audit is a necessary part of evidence-based practice. Once the evidence has been gathered from national, regional, local and professional sources, appraised for validity and applicability to your clinical situation, and implemented as best practice, clinical audit is employed to determine whether best practice is occurring on a day-to-day basis (NHS Executive, 1998a). Without this measurement process, a vital link in determining the impact of evidence-based practice on patient care is lost (the word 'patient' is intended to include all clients or users of health services). Without audit, you simply do not know whether what you are doing is working as intended.

This chapter seeks to give a simple, straightforward account of the auditing process to assist you in carrying out your own audits. We will guide you through the audit process and provide insights gained from our experience in conducting clinical audit. After reading this chapter you will be able to conduct a clinical audit by following the key stages of the audit process (National Centre for Clinical Audit, 1997):

- Decide on the topic to audit, the reason for doing the audit, how the quality of service is going to be measured in the audit and the cases to be included.
- Collect data on practice using the agreed measures.
- Evaluate the findings to identify any shortcomings in care and their causes.
- Act to make improvements in care.
- Repeat the data collection, evaluation and action steps as often as needed to achieve and sustain improvement.

WHAT IS CLINICAL AUDIT?

Clinical audit is a clinically led initiative which seeks to improve the quality and outcome of patient care through structured peer review whereby clinicians examine their practices and results against agreed explicit standards and modify their practice where indicated (NHS Executive, 1996). Audit is therefore a systematic comparison against an agreed standard, derived from the available evidence and agreed by clinical professionals. (The word 'clinician' or 'clinical professional' is intended to include physicians, nurses, midwives, health visitors, professions allied to medicine and any other member of the healthcare team with patient care responsibilities.) Audit provides confirmation of the consistent application of best practice, or reveals practice that is inconsistent and ineffective. Audit is a cyclical process which results in action to change undesirable practice or maintain good practice.

Audit has moved on from being merely a mechanism used to review and monitor standards of care. It no longer only examines records retrospectively but increasingly embraces concurrent and electronic audit. Initially medical and nursing audits were carried out separately but more recently organisations have established clinical audit which recognises the multidisciplinary contribution to patient outcomes. It measures what the client receives from all internal and external providers of care.

WHAT CLINICAL AUDIT IS NOT

Clinical audit is not a resource management tool, although audit findings often inform resource decisions. Audit findings may uncover areas where savings can be made, but may also highlight the need to add resources.

Additional resources, usually time and money, may be needed to carry out training or buy equipment. Avoid the temptation to use clinical audit strictly to inform resource decision making. The intent of clinical audit is to measure and improve care. Resource implications, although important, should never be the driver for clinical audit.

Clinical audit should never be used to threaten an individual clinician suspected of poor practice. Audit is, in itself, a neutral measurement process. Ideally, all clinical professionals on your service or unit should be involved in agreeing the topic for the audit and the cases to be reviewed. The use of clinical audit as a weapon to expose poorly performing clinicians will result in resistance to audit and, potentially, to sabotage of the audit process. Audit findings must be handled confidentially and sensitively when poor individual performance is identified (NHS Executive, 1998a).

Clinical audit is not a batch of expensive computers or a set of complicated statistics. Audit is a process that involves design, measurement, evaluation, and action to make corrections or maintain good performance. Audit often requires observation of care either directly or by review of the clinical notes, which is largely a process that requires people, not machines. As we move towards an electronic medical record designed to allow us to extract details of care, electronic audit will become more common. For now, most audits are completed using simple comparisons, and findings are reported in percentages of compliance with the standard.

Clinical audit is not about competition between clinical professionals. There is a temptation to compare audit findings across groups and make judgements about 'good' and 'bad' professionals based on the results. This competition misses the point. Audit is about improving patient care and ensuring consistent application of standards in practice. This requires clinical professionals to measure their care against the standards, not each other.

WHO BENEFITS FROM CLINICAL AUDIT?

Since clinical audit contributes to clinically effective care, the main beneficiaries of the clinical audit process should be the patients. Patient expectations have increased with the introduction of policy innovations such as the 'Patients Charter'. Litigation and complaints have increased as patients' expectations rise. A more knowledgeable and demanding patient population is seeking more assurances that clinical care is effective and safe. The public increasingly expect evidence of implementation of the latest advances in medical care and technology. Contract purchasers (such as health authorities or general practitioner groups) often seek audit information as evidence of the provision of quality services as outlined by the purchaser's specifications of service required. A vigorous and well-informed audit programme supports good clinical decision making and can provide evidence that best practice is in place and working to benefit patients.

In addition to benefiting the patient through improved care, audit can support teamwork and learning in the clinical area. Arnold *et al.*, (1992) suggested that a unit or practice with a variety of audit topics in progress has cohesiveness and team spirit that is often missing in complacent or less well organised settings. Clinical professionals are genuinely concerned about the quality of care they give both individually and collectively. Audit is often the first step in providing evidence for and about practice and serves as a baseline from which improvements in care can be made. Clinical audit involves groups of people, often from different disciplines, agreeing topics and approaches to audit. This collaboration through audit can build a common purpose and focus. The process of clinical audit builds skills and experience for the team members involved. Feedback from audit activities can suggest areas for further development of clinical skills and knowledge that supports educational planning.

Audit findings can also support the financial and resource decisions of an organisation. For example, an audit of ambulation protocols after hip surgery may reveal that the protocols are implemented more consistently during the week when therapy and nursing staffing levels are higher. These findings could suggest that a revision of staffing levels over the weekend may improve compliance with the standard. Audits conducted of dressing change practices may find that expensive specialty dressing materials are being used when lower-cost dressing supplies are just as effective for the clinical situation. Both examples have resource implications, one situation suggesting where resources need to be added and another where money can be saved. Maximising your resources can save time, money and result in better client care.

Audit may be the only way of justifying investments in new services. It could materially increase your power to bargain for additional resources (Arnold *et al.*, 1992).

IS AUDIT THE SAME AS RESEARCH?

Clinical audit and research are not the same, although they both contribute to improving the effectiveness of clinical practice. Research is used to define good practice, whereas audit measures the extent to which good practice (as defined through research and expert opinion) is implemented on a daily basis. Observation or data collection to determine current practice is another form of information gathering which is sometimes used alongside research and audit. Each activity has a role to play in clinically effective care (NHS Executive, 1998b).

If a group of clinicians was to set out to determine what is best practice in a given clinical area, the first step would be to search the literature and other sources (see Chapter 3) for what has been discovered through research. Some areas of clinical practice have a growing research base (such as wound care and breastfeeding), whereas others have few published research findings. If the published research is sparse, there may be well-documented expert opinion on which to base best practice. In the absence of research or expert opinion, the group could choose to design and conduct a research study, perhaps in collaboration with the local university.

On occasion, clinicians may be faced with determining what practice is actually occurring in their area. This requires neither research nor clinical audit. This situation requires a structured observation or data collection to determine the variety and frequency of different types of practice. For example, nurses working in cancer services may be interested in what complementary therapies are used to support pain management in their hospice care. Investigating this might include reviewing notes and interviewing nurses and other clinical professionals to catalogue which therapies they use. The data collection does not attempt to compare the effectiveness of one therapy with another; it simply intends to list the approaches used and perhaps describe the relative popularity of various practices.

Once best practice has been implemented, clinical audit is used to evaluate how practice meets those standards. Audit aims to review current practice by using existing knowledge and to improve patient care in the practice setting. It usually relates to a particular practice or unit (although it can have a broader base such as a regional audit) with the intention of providing feedback to those involved. It is about testing the application of knowledge, not about discovering knowledge. Audit is an ongoing process which tests and retests practice against standards.

To assist you in selecting the most appropriate approach, guidelines are suggested in Box 7.1 (NHS Executive, 1998b).

Box 7.1 Guidelines for the evaluation of practice

Research is appropriate when:
◆ best practice is not defined through existing research or expert opinion
◆ comparisons are needed to determine the best patient outcomes resulting from differing practices.

Data collection or structured observation is appropriate when:
◆ practice patterns are unknown
◆ the intent of the observation is to catalogue prevailing practice patterns without making judgements about appropriateness or effectiveness.

Clinical audit is appropriate when:
◆ best practice is defined and has been implemented
◆ the intent is to determine consistency of practice with the agreed standard.

Avoid the temptation to be less meticulous in your approach to audit because you do not see it as research. Adopt a thorough approach to design, procedure, analysis and interpretation of your findings. Rigour in designing and conducting audit lends credibility to the findings and supports good clinical decision making.

THE CLINICAL AUDIT PROCESS

Figure 7.1 depicts the process for clinical audit suggested by the National Centre for Clinical Audit (1997a). By taking each step in turn, we will explore how this process can be accomplished in your setting.

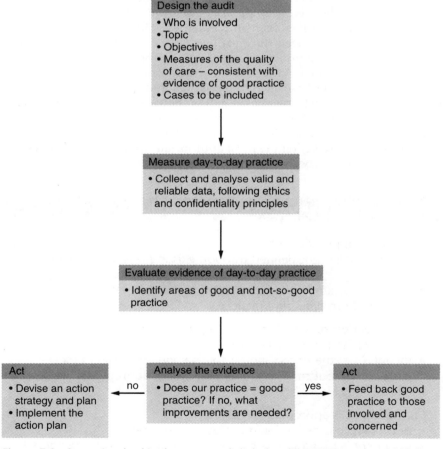

Figure 7.1 Stages involved in the process of clinical audit (NHS Executive, 1998a).

Key stage 1: Designing the audit

Who is involved?

Ideally, all clinicians who have a stake in the service provided should be involved in selecting the topics for clinical audit (NHS Executive, 1998a). This means that consultation with physicians, nurses and other clinical professionals is recommended to agree the topic. The consultation process will build support for the audit and you will gain valuable insights into what aspects of clinical care the team is most concerned about or interested in exploring. During this design phase, it is important to gain the commitment of clinical professionals to potentially changing their practice if the evidence gathered by audit supports this. Without this commitment, clinical audit can be a time-wasting and frustrating experience.

You may wish to put together a clinical audit team who will assist you with the design and conduct of the audit. Working as part of a dynamic team provides a rewarding environment for the development of standards of practice and audits. A team also facilitates a positive exchange of ideas and information among colleagues and across disciplines. Although the team designs and conducts the audit collectively, it may be useful to appoint team members into these roles:

1. **Audit leader** The audit leader should to be the same person through-out the project. Try to choose someone who has experience in your practice area and, ideally, someone with experience in clinical audit. The leader's role is to guide and coordinate the audit team, and to ensure the audit is conducted following the principles of ethics and confidentiality.

2. **Liaison with the audit committee** If your organisation has a clinical audit committee, one of your team members should be appointed to communicate and consult with the audit committee. This liaison role can tap into the expertise of the audit committee and save time in designing and conducting your study. Audit committees are usually set up in organisations to consider proposals by practitioners who wish to implement specific audits. They also control funding, coordinate audit activity across the organisation and review particular topics.

3. **Team members** All members of your audit team should be willing to assist in communicating with their peers, reviewing evidence, participating in data collection, and developing action plans for areas of improvement. Team members must agree to observe confidentiality and respect the potentially sensitive nature of the findings. A commitment to improving patient care is essential.

4. **Other useful supports to the team** Other clinical professionals in your organisation may have experience in audit and be willing to share

their experiences. Be open to the internal consultancy they can bring. Your local university may be willing to provide assistance in searching the literature or designing the study. Information on clinical audit is available through books, pamphlets (see reference list) and on the Internet. Do not limit yourself: there is lots of information available.

Using an audit team enhances the educational aspects of audit. The teamwork supports a useful exchanges of ideas, information and opinions within the group.

What is the topic?

The team of clinical professionals in your area is usually the best source of topics for clinical audit. Clinicians are often aware of innovations in practice through reading and networking and are interested in how they measure up against best practice. People working on your team are also closest to patients' experiences and can provide information on how practices impact the patient. The key to choosing an audit topic is to choose something that really matters to the patient and that the clinicians agree they can do something about. For example, there may be a standard (perhaps built into an integrated care pathway) that elderly patients admitted with pneumonia will be discharged home in 1 week. This standard clearly matters to the patient and has implications for care. In order to be discharged in 1 week, presumably the pneumonia must be resolving, and the patient must be able to manage at home. This means the care in hospital must be designed to maintain or improve strength, mobility, nutrition and independence while treating the underlying pneumonia. This would be an excellent topic for clinical audit since planning care that maximises fitness at discharge is clearly under the control of the team.

However, we have seen clinicians undertake clinical audit of topics over which those professionals have little control. A classic example of this is when a hospital conducts a patient satisfaction survey asking patients what they think of the decor in the wards. If there is no money or intention of improving the decor, then don't ask. Asking people for their opinions sends the message that you are interested and willing to take action. If you don't take action, you have, in their minds, broken a promise.

Prioritising topics for audit can be a challenge. Clinical professionals in your team may have differing views of what really matters to the patient. Box 7.2 gives a tried and tested list of suggestions for deciding what to audit.

Avoid the temptation to audit only the things you are doing well. Once you are consistently meeting your standard, look for something that you can improve.

Box 7.2 Deciding what to audit

High-risk practices High-risk practices are those actions that, if done poorly, could result in serious consequences for the patient. Many technical aspects of care fall into this category such as medication protocols, cardiac monitoring, invasive procedures, conscious sedation and emergency psychiatric assessment.

High-volume practices These are the types of care that you do a lot of and, because they are common practice, can affect many patients. For example, midwives who give family planning advice after childbirth potentially affect hundreds of families. If the advice is unclear, inconsistent or misunderstood, the patient may be compromised. Auditing this type of care could result in the development of family planning materials in languages other than English or potentially in the use of culturally based patient advocates to support the midwives' advice.

High-cost care Many clinical professionals dislike considering the cost of care in making clinical decisions; unfortunately, the realities of limited budgets has opened the discussion. Audits of high-cost care do not always result in demands to reduce costs; they can, in fact, support the need for continued spending. For example, a standard may have been set that a postoperative patient may need special respiratory treatments because the practice results in fewer cases of pneumonia and quicker discharge. Auditing this practice to gather evidence that supports the continued high-cost treatments is important.

Topics of local concern As mentioned above, the clinical professionals working in your area are the best source of topics for audit based on their professional knowledge and experience of patient care. Several other local sources should also be considered. Your Trust or service may become concerned about a patient care practice in response to complaints or adverse events uncovered through risk management activities. For example, your complaints officer may bring to your attention a complaint that an elderly patient did not receive needed assistance with eating while a patient on your ward. Since your standard of care clearly identifies that staff will assess nutritional status and develop a plan for supporting nutritional deficit when identified, you may conduct an audit to determine whether the failure in this case was an isolated event or a trend requiring more comprehensive action.

Objectives

Your Trust may require you to write a proposal before conducting your audit, or you may have a more informal mechanism for communicating audit plans and activities (such as through completing a form). Either way, it is a good idea to decide and record the objectives of your audit. Objectives keep you focused on the goal, that is, the positive intention of the audit. The objectives of an audit study should include the benefit for the patient. Usually the objective is to ensure good practice or to improve care. Be specific about the topic to be audited (NHS Executive, 1998a). Some examples may be: 'The audit is intended to ensure consistent application of the teaching standards for family planning advice adopted 6 months ago' or 'The audit is designed to measure effective management of discharge to home'. Keeping the objective focused on patient care will avoid the trap of 'navel gazing', that is, examining clinical practice for its own sake without attention to patient outcomes.

Identifying measures of quality consistent with good practice

The next step in designing a clinical audit is to state clearly the specific measures you will use in your study. You should have some sort of standards of care in place in your unit, otherwise you have no agreed baseline from which to conduct the audit. You may be basing your standards on guidance from your professional body, a governmental agency (National Service Framework), expert opinion (found in professional journals and text-books), or on research. However, standards must be evaluated and tailored to your situation, and agreed by the clinical professionals doing the work. For the purposes of conducting an audit, standards should be in writing (such as in the audit proposal) and easily understood by every team member. This keeps the audit process collaborative and open, supporting the intention to improve patient care. It is important that your audit team makes the final decisions about the standards to be audited against.

Grimshaw and Russell (1993) describe standards of care as:

> *Authoritative statements of (a) minimum levels of acceptable performance or results, or (b) excellent levels of performance or results, or (c) the range of acceptable performance or results.*

Standards of care should be reviewed periodically to ensure they are still consistent with good practice and your situation. Standards often need review when new services or new technology are added. For example, the introduction of thrombolytic therapy in the treatment of early myocardial infarction required new standards of assessment and early diagnosis in accident and emergency departments to maximise the benefit of the therapy.

If you are involved in developing your own standards, you are more likely to implement any resulting changes. Setting standards locally can play an important part in the success of the audit.

In order to use standards of care in a clinical audit, it is necessary to turn them into indicators. Indicators are developed from the standards of care and they are usually specific to your area of practice. The National Centre for Clinical Audit (1997b) provides this definition of an indicator:

> *Quantitative statements which are used to measure quality of care. Indicators always include a percentage, ratio or other quantitative way of saying how many patients the expected care should be provided for.*

The indicator states the level of compliance it requires to ensure the standard of care. If your standard is that all patients receive medication teaching before discharge, then the indicator level is probably appropriately set at 100%. However, some patients are not candidates for medication teaching because of dementia or other impairment. Perhaps it is more appropriate to exclude patients with dementia from the audit sample, or to modify the indicator so that 100% of patients *or their designated carers* will receive medication teaching before discharge. Be sure your indicator reflects a reasonable interpretation of your standard of care (Table 7.1).

Reflection   What standards of care are in place in your area of practice? Are they evidence-based and current? When were your standards of care last reviewed and revised to include new knowledge?

   Choose several standards of care and turn them into indicators. How did you decide what quantitative measure (percentage) to use in your indicator and why? Do your peers agree with the quantitative measures you have chosen?

Cases to be included

The final step in designing a clinical audit is to decide what cases are to be included in the study. The decision is made based on the objectives of the audit. If the objective is to see whether a new practice introduced 6 months previously has been consistently implemented, the cases chosen for

Table 7.1 Examples of standards of care and indicators	
Standard of Care	**Indicator**
Children under 2 years old are immunised against tetanus and polio	90% of 2 year olds immunised against tetanus and polio
The notes of clients sensitive to penicillin are clearly marked	The notes of all (100%) clients sensitive to penicillin are clearly marked
The incidence of wound infections in postoperative clients is reduced	Wound infections are reduced to less than 5% in all postoperative clients

review should be limited to the last 6 months. If the objective is to compare current practice to a newly developed (and as yet unimplemented practice) as a baseline evaluation, you may wish to include only cases from the last month.

Deciding the numbers of cases to include can be problematic. If the topic to be audited is a high-risk but low-volume procedure (such as intra-aortic balloon pump management), you may wish to include all cases. If, on the other hand, the practice is frequent, you may wish to include a small sample to keep the data manageable. Research and statistics textbooks offer guidelines for sampling to ensure reliability and generalisability in research studies, although it is probably not necessary to go to these sources to design a good clinical audit. Your audit department can help you with deciding these matters if you need help. Generally, if you keep the objectives in mind and consult with the clinicians involved in the care of the patients, you will design a meaningful study.

Pulling it all together: examples of clinical audit designs

Two examples of designs for clinical audit are given. Audit 1 concerns pain management in an orthopaedic clinic; audit 2 looks at patient non-attendance at a dementia clinic for the elderly.

The pain management audit below is an example of a retrospective audit, which means the audit looks back over cases that have occurred

---

Example: Audit 1 – Pain management

A group of clinicians is concerned that pain management in their orthopaedic clinic is not as effective as it could be. Some patients have required admission to hospital for intensive treatment of back pain. Standards are in place that include assessment of pain using a rating scale at each visit and implementation of a variety of techniques for reports of pain.

An audit team was formed with members from various disciplines. The topic was discussed with the nurses, therapists and consultants in the clinic who were involved in the care of patients with chronic back pain. It was agreed that the audit would be valuable, and an openness to changing practice was voiced.

The audit team identified the following objective for the study: 'This audit is intended to ensure the effective management of pain in patients attending the orthopaedic clinic.'

The audit team reviewed the current standards of care and turned them into indicators.

Example: Audit 1 – Cont'd

Standards of care	Indicators
On admission to the clinic, all patients will be assessed for pain	100% of patients will have a pain assessment at the first visit using a 10-point scale
All patients reporting significant pain will receive instruction on visualisation or other pain control techniques	100% of patients reporting 4 or above on the 10-point scale will receive instruction on a pain control technique at that visit
Patients previously taught a pain control technique will be reassessed for pain level and effectiveness of the technique	100% of patients taught a pain control technique will be reassessed using the 10-point scale at the next visit

It was decided to include all patients admitted to the orthopaedic clinic for chronic back pain in the last 3 months.

Example: Audit 2 – Failure to attend follow-up appointments

A group of clinicians became concerned when the patient non-attendance rate at their elderly dementia clinic began to climb. There were standards in place to address non-attendance including appointment reminders and flexible transportation arrangements.

An audit team was assembled including a clerk who does some of the appointment scheduling and nurses who coordinate contact with the caregivers.

The objective of the audit was: 'To improve patient attendance rate at follow-up visits'.

Standards of care	Indicators
Patients are advised of their follow-up appointment within 5 days of the consultation	100% of patient appointment letters are sent within 5 days of the consultation
Transportation needs are assessed at each visit	100% of patients have their transportation needs assessed at each visit

Example: Audit 2 – Cont'd

Reminder cards are posted 7 days before the next follow-up visit	100% of reminder cards are posted 7 days before the appointment date
Caregivers are instructed to call the clinic to reschedule if the patient cannot attend the appointment	100% of caregivers will reschedule if the patient is unable to attend

The audit team decided to include all cases where there was non-attendance over the next 3 months.

in the past. Retrospective audits are often more easily managed as the audit team can plan a time to sit down and collect data from case notes or other sources. The disadvantage of retrospective audits is that there is no opportunity to make an improvement in care for those patients.

The dementia clinic audit was designed as a concurrent study, which is one that examines cases as they occur. Concurrent studies give you the opportunity to make corrections in substandard care as it arises. The staff in the dementia clinic were clearly concerned about ensuring the patients received the necessary follow-up care, so a concurrent audit was suggested. Both designs are useful ways to gather data for audit purposes.

Key stage 2: Measure day-to-day practice

Gathering data

The next step in the audit process is the collection and analysis of valid and reliable data following ethics and confidentiality principles (National Centre for Clinical Audit, 1997a). Many sources of data are potentially useful for audit purposes, including any documentation used for the provision and delivery of care. It is imperative that confidentiality of patient information be ensured during the audit process. Patient names should never be recorded on data collection sheets. If it is necessary to track the patients included in the study, a coding system should be designed to preserve anonymity, perhaps by recording the patient record number. Similarly, data collected on the practice patterns of an individual professional should not be identifiable. All members of the audit team need to agree and respect these principles during the audit process.

Some examples of data sources used in clinical audit are:

1. **Patient records** Mobility assessments, neurological signs, advice on lifting, analgesic prescriptions, referrals to medical specialists, referrals to other specialist healthcare professionals, care plans, diaries, health visitor records, admission notes, social service records, social workers records, Kardex.

2. **Registers** Child health, Family Health Services Authority (FHSA) (age/sex), cancer register, diagnostic index, social services preferred provider (Blue book).

3. **Computer information or other organisational records** Patient administration system, clinical coding department, Korner data, district statistics, financial information, case-mix system, resource management, risk management, committee reports, adverse events reports, legal action, complaints.

The data collection tools used in a successful audit have to be simple and repeatable so that data can be gathered continually using the chosen format. You need to discuss the different types of tools that can be used and devise one that best suits your purpose. Types of tools include checklists, observations and questionnaires.

Checklists. Checklists are useful when you are collecting data from patient records or other documents. The checklist should be designed to record the data described by the indicator. For example, if you were designing a checklist to use in auditing patient records in the pain management example above, the checklist would probably take the form of a statement followed by a 'yes' or 'no' column for the data collector to record the findings. Statements should reflect the indicator clearly so that there is no confusion. Examples of statements for the pain management audit could be:

Pain assessment completed at first visit	Yes	No
If pain rating above 4, pain control technique taught	Yes	No
Type of technique taught..		
Pain reassessed on next visit	Yes	No

Observations. Observation of practice is another data collection technique. Data collectors record their observations and the findings are analysed. Often an observation record is designed to assist the data collector to record the events quickly and consistently. Sometimes audio or video recordings are made, or data are gathered from monitor tapes, computer files or other machine-generated sources.

Questionnaires. Questionnaires are useful for gathering information from people. Questionnaires may be used to guide an interview or may be designed for the person to fill in and return to the data collector. The questions should be clear and unambiguous, asking for only one piece of information per question. For example, the question, 'Did you receive your reminder card before your appointment?' can be answered decisively with a yes or no. However, the question, 'Were your meals attractively presented and tasty?' asks two separate questions which may have conflicting answers.

Analysing the data

Once the data are collected, they must be analysed and presented in a way that allows them to be compared with the standard. Most audit findings are reported as percentage compliance with the standard, often with explanatory notes.

In the pain management audit example, the findings would probably look something like the example shown below.

Analysis can sometimes be challenging. The above findings suggest that pain assessment is more consistently conducted on the first visit. However,

---

Example: Audit 1 – Pain management findings

The audit was conducted by reviewing the clinical notes of 46 patients referred for chronic back pain who attended as new cases to the clinic between 1 January and 30 June.

Indicator	Findings
100% of patients will have a pain assessment at the first visit using a 10-point scale	92% of records reviewed had documentation of a pain assessment
100% of patients reporting 4 or above on the 10-point scale will receive instruction on a pain control technique at that visit	67% of records reviewed had documentation of instruction on a pain control technique **Note** An additional 7% of notes recorded refusal of instruction; a further 12% were non-English-speaking patients
100% of patients taught a pain control technique will be reassessed using a 10-point scale at the next visit	72% of records reviewed had documentation of reassessment at the next visit

the audit team knows that the findings from the initial visit are recorded on a detailed assessment form which specifically asks for the results of the pain scale, whereas the follow-up visits are recorded as notes. Is the difference between compliance on the first visit and subsequent visits due to ease of recording rather than not doing the assessment? Often the findings raise further issues such as, 'Was there any information as to why the patients refused instruction?' or 'Were there any non-English-speaking patients who received instruction, and how?'. It is these discussions among the audit team and the clinical professionals involved that are of real value in analysing the audit findings.

Key stage 3: Evaluate evidence of day-to-day practice

Once the audit findings have been analysed and the resulting questions explored, a decision is made as to whether day-to-day practice represents good practice. Crombie and Davies (1993) suggested that the explanation for lack of success in improving the quality in healthcare is due to the omission of a vital step of the process. They proposed that the missing link is the step that identifies *why* current practice fails to meet the required standard. They suggested that it is not sufficient to establish that a problem exists, or even to describe it in detail. Once a problem has been identified, the underlying causes need to be sought and understood. Solving the problem should then be possible.

In our pain management audit, the team decided to explore the findings with clinical professionals who care for the patients. In the discussions with staff, it was discovered that clinicians were not necessarily conducting pain assessments using the 10-point rating scale. The nurses reported that, if the patient was making remarks about feeling well and looked comfortable, they did not conduct a structured pain assessment. It was also discovered that many non-English-speaking patients were already using complementary therapies for pain management, so the staff were not teaching them any new ones.

Based on these discussions, the audit team decided that the staff were exercising appropriate clinical judgement not to teach additional complementary therapies to patients already using them, but they were concerned that, contrary to the research in pain management, staff were assuming that patients were pain free because they failed to display certain behaviours associated with acute pain such as grimacing and moaning.

Audit results are seldom as clearcut as in our example. Audit teams will find that situations sometimes cloud the decision. When a clinical area has low morale, high workloads or an influx of new staff members, the audit findings may demonstrate less compliance. This may be a self-correcting problem or it may need action for improvement. Audit teams often find themselves weighing the findings carefully and gathering more data before deciding. This is particularly important when serious inconsistencies are discovered or individual practice patterns are questionable.

Key stage 4: Take action

If the audit team comes to the decision that the results of the audit are consistent with good practice, it is important that feedback reaches the clinical professionals involved. When good practice is celebrated, it tends to be continued.

When the decision is made that practice could be improved, it is essential to involve the staff in determining the action plan to overcome the problems. People are more likely to carry through a plan of correction that they designed than one that is imposed. Make a detailed action plan, complete with deadlines, which describes how the situation will be corrected (NHS Executive, 1998a).

Action plans for correction can contain many strategies. Here are some common solutions:

1. **Education** Education is the solution only when ignorance is the problem. Before you assume that people need a training session on a particular skill, check it out. Ask people what they know, or watch them perform the skill to see whether it is up to standard. Training people who are already knowledgeable or proficient is a waste of time.

2. **Change the system** People sometimes fail to meet standards because they cannot easily access the information, supplies or assistance they need. Perhaps the paperwork is getting in the way or the team is not communicating effectively. Find out what is stopping people from performing to standard and correct that.

3. **Correct behaviour** It is sometimes necessary to address poor performance directly. You may find yourself pursuing a disciplinary proceeding, but this is uncommon. If you are unsure what to do about an individual staff member, get help from your manager or director of human resources.

Praise good practice and correct poor practice. Blame has no place in the action plan for improvement.

Key stage 5: Repeat the audit cycle

Too often a plan of improvement is designed and implemented, but the audit is never repeated to determine the effect. Repeat the data collection shortly after the changes have been implemented to see whether improvement has occurred (NHS Executive, 1998a). If there is improvement, remember to feedback to your team and praise the accomplishment. If there is no improvement, you may not have discovered the cause of the problem, or the action plan for correction was inaccurate. Review the findings, explore your decisions and try again.

Now it's your turn...

Have you thought about your own audit project? Consider an aspect of service provision or patient care within your organisation which you could audit. Examples include the following:

- patients' understanding of their condition
- patient satisfaction
- readmission rates, non-attendance, access to service
- meeting targets for immunisation or screening
- infection rates and methods of infection control
- child protection issues
- effectiveness of a particular practice such as management of hypoglycaemia in diabetic patients or wound care
- integrated care pathways.

Reflection   Having considered the audit process it is useful to reflect upon what you have learned so far. Write down possible audit topics and an appropriate objective.

Topic examples	Objective
• Access to, or satisfaction with, service	
• Relevance to need	
• Effectiveness	
• Efficiency and economy	
• High-risk care	

Audit plan

You are now ready to start your own audit process by making a plan. Your plan will be useful in the preparation of your audit proposal which will be submitted to your managers and to the clinical audit team within your organisation. The audit plan should include the following:

- Who is involved (include audit team)?
- What is the topic and why?
- What are the objectives?
- What are the measures of the quality of care (standards and indicators)?
- Which cases are to be included (types, numbers, concurrent or retrospective)?

- How will the data be collected (do we need to develop a questionnaire or other tool)?
- How will ethical and confidential treatment of the data be ensured?

CHALLENGES WITHIN THE AUDIT PROCESS

Although there are many benefits to conducting clinical audit, there are some challenges to be considered. There is a risk that audit could be perceived as policing. Donabidian (1992), one of the major figures in quality improvement in healthcare, acknowledges that the audit process can be misused, as can every other form of human endeavour. It can be used to stifle individuality and creativity in practice. However, audit can be used as a constructive activity that is intended to recognise and reward good work and to improve morale, by allowing people to examine what they do. In turn practitioners become self-governing, self-correcting and self-disciplining rather than being the subject of control by external agencies. Clinical audit empowers nurses, doctors and other professionals to observe their own activities using analytical tools, to become enthusiastic about new discoveries, and to be recognised and respected as people who achieve high standards.

Many people may view audit as yet another burden to add to their already busy professional roles. They believe that they do not have the time. Audit is a waste of time only if it is not done properly. Efficiently managed and implemented audit can indicate time-saving measures and support change. However, change can occur only after properly conducted enquiry and evaluation.

ACCOUNTABILITY AND THE AUDIT PROCESS

The statutory obligation for quality has been added to the duties of the chief executives of NHS Trusts (Department of Health, 1998). Clinical audit is likely to be one of the components of a comprehensive approach to ensuring clinical effectiveness in NHS organisations. Although the chief executive may have ultimate accountability for audit in a legal sense, it is the clinical professionals within the organisation who must use their experience and judgement to determine standards, and to design and conduct meaningful audit studies. It is those same professionals who in turn must implement improvements in care consistent with best practice as it evolves. Clinical professionals are accountable for their decisions and actions. Clinical audit is one way for clinicians to demonstrate integrity and ownership of the responsibilities for safe and effective care. We challenge you to develop your skill in audit, and to make the ongoing evaluation of your care a priority.

REFERENCES

Arnold, C., Brain, J., Brown, R., Horden, R., Laidlaw, J., McAleer, S. & Wood, R. (1992). *Moving to Audit. What Every Doctor Needs to Know About Medical Audit.* Dundee: Centre for Medical Education, University of Dundee.

Crombie, L. & Davies, H. (1993). Missing link in the audit cycle. *Quality in Health Care,* **2,** 47–48.

Department of Health (1997). *The New NHS: Modern, Dependable.* London: HMSO.

Donabidian, A. Cited in Dolan, B. (1992). A legend in his own lifetime. *Nursing Standard,* **7**(9), 20–21.

Grimshaw, J. & Russell, I. (1993). Achieving health gain through clinical guidelines. I: Developing scientifically valid guidelines. *Quality in Health Care,* **2,** 243–248.

Luthert, J. & Robinson, L. (eds) (1993). *The Royal Marsden Hospital Manual of Standards of Care.* Oxford: Blackwell.

National Centre for Clinical Audit (1997a). *Key Points from Audit Literature Related to Criteria for Clinical Audit.* London: NCCA.

National Centre for Clinical Audit (1997b). *Glossary of Terms Used in NCCA Criteria for Clinical Audit.* London: NCCA.

NHS Executive (1996). *Clinical Audit in the NHS. Using Clinical Audit in the NHS: A Position Statement.* Leeds: NHS Executive.

NHS Executive (1998a). *Achieving Effective Practice. A Clinical Effectiveness and Research Information Pack for Nurses, Midwives and Health Visitors. 5: Designing and Carrying Out an Audit.* Leeds: NHS Executive.

NHS Executive (1998b). *Achieving Effective Practice. A Clinical Effectiveness and Research Information Pack for Nurses, Midwives and Health Visitors. 6: Preparing a Proposal for Clinical Audit.* Leeds: NHS Executive.

3

Section 3

Reflecting Upon the Evidence

Personal change

Bryce Taylor

KEY ISSUES

◆ Finding the time

◆ Believing it is possible to make a difference

◆ Getting out of the habit – whatever the habit is

◆ Where do I go from here?

◆ How did I get here at all?

◆ Where else can I go?

◆ Is there any point in even thinking about alternatives when there is so much to manage?

Having found and appraised sources of evidence, and decided on an implemention strategy, we often find that our plans go somewhat adrift. Colleagues do not agree or seem to construct barriers to progress. Maybe we feel personally overwhelmed or the organisation itself is so stretched that we begin to observe poor practice. In this final section of the book, authors address personal, ethical and organisational aspects of change.

THE PRESSURES OF WORK

How many of the following apply to the work you do?

• Insufficient training to meet the demands of the role
• Insufficient preparation for the future
• Insufficient supervision about the issues arising in the work
• Pressure to do more with less and do it less well

- Role overload and role conflict
- Unsatisfactory working conditions
- Too long hours
- Too little variation in the range of the work
- Lack of material recognition (e.g. too little pay)
- Inadequate or uncertain levels of funding or resourcing to do the job well
- A sense that those served appreciate your efforts less and less
- 'Political' constraints that inhibit individual initiative
- A gap between aspiration and accomplishment
- The lack of a strategic plan, purpose or direction in the management of the agency.

Many of us know the feeling of 'overwhelm' that comes with knowing things will not get better unless we do something else – something more.

For most of us that realisation comes as yet another burden. Just when we want some relief, some answer to it all, we have to wake up to the fact that there is no answer and that any remedies not only lie in our own hands, but will be found only by creating the time in addition to all else we are having to carry. Some of the burden is a result of our personal myths – exaggerated or unrealistic beliefs we have about ourselves, the situation or other people. Some of the ideas that are particularly strong in the helping professions at the present time include the following:

1. It is a dire necessity for a helping professional to be loved or appreciated by every client.
2. You must always enjoy the favour of your superviser.
3. You must be thoroughly competent and successful in doing your job if you are to consider yourself worthwhile.
4. Anyone who disagrees with your ideas and methods is 'bad' and becomes an opponent to be scorned or rejected.
5. You should become very upset over clients' problems and failings.
6. It is awful and catastrophic when clients and the institution do not behave as you would like them to.
7. Your unhappiness is caused by clients or the institution and you have little or no ability to control your emotional reactions.
8. Until clients and the institution straighten themselves out and do what is right, you have no responsibility to do what is right yourself.
9. There is invariably a right, precise and perfect solution to human problems and it is catastrophic if that solution is not found (Edelwich and Brodsky, 1980).

DOING SOMETHING ABOUT IT

Of course, doing something about all this is dangerous, especially if it works and makes a difference, because then we begin to realise that we can influence events in however small a way; so beware of the next step which is:

- Write down a seemingly insoluble work-related problem – any problem that you feel strongly as your own. For example, 'One of my co-workers speaks to clients in a high-handed, patronising way which lowers their self-esteem and undermines my efforts to help them'. Then 'brainstorm' and write down all the alternative solutions you can think of. Do not try to evaluate any of them at this stage. You will not be able to think of many solutions if you let the 'red-pencil mentality' edit them out before you get them down on paper.

When you have exhausted your brainstorming capacity, you can evaluate all the alternatives by putting each into one of the categories shown in Box 8.1.

One of the immediate benefits of this exercise, before a solution is even decided upon, is simply to show how often the thing that is going to happen anyway is about the worst thing that can happen. You do not know what the outcome will be if you try to do something about the problem. But you can be pretty sure of the outcome if you do nothing, namely, no change.

Box 8.1 Categorisation of alternative solutions to a problem

1. Most likely Other things being equal, what do you think will happen? Usually the answer is: 'I will go on complaining, and nothing will change'.

2. Most desirable This is the 'magic wand' solution, where you can indulge in any fantasy, for example: 'The offending party will disappear from the face of the earth'.

3. More than a 50/50 chance of success An example here might be: 'I will write a memorandum to the director documenting my co-worker's unprofessional conduct'.

4. Less than a 50/50 chance of success Here you might list some remedies that have been tried previously without success, such as 'I will have to talk with my errant co-worker about the harm he/she is doing'.

5. Least desirable This might be: 'I will criticise my co-worker publicly, thus causing him/her to retaliate in such a way as to damage my professional reputation'. Or: 'I will give up on the situation and quit my job'. Or it might simply be the same as the 'most likely' solution: 'I will do nothing, and things will stay the same'.

Tactical responses

The timing of a response can play an important part in determining the difference it is likely to make, so bear in mind the stage that fits best:

1. **Enthusiasm–realism** This is the best time for intervention – before the damage is done.
2. **Stagnation–movement** At this stage further education and other interventions designed to get a stalled career going again are especially useful.
3. **Frustration–satisfaction** In this stage the energy of discontent creates the possibility of change.
4. **Apathy–involvement** If a person cares enough to be disappointed, is there a way to turn that feeling around?

For many of us, the addition of a personal crisis can add an extra dimension to a situation that has been managed (just) and now it is at breaking point. Many people working in contemporary organisations realise the degree to which they drive themselves only when something unpleasant makes them stop in their tracks; they then experience the full impact of their exhaustion. For many of us, knowing what we might do to help ourselves is anything but a guarantee that we will act in time or with the kind of compassion for ourselves that we extend to others.

So this chapter begins with the author recognising that it is one thing to talk about how better to manage personal change and another for the reader to find the time for all the suggestions that it might contain. So, as much as anything, this chapter provides frameworks for thinking about change, and is offered as a resource to return to rather than to be read and forgotten.

ATTITUDES AND APPROACHES TO CHANGE

Change can be approached from different directions. There are changes we wish for, changes we initiate and promote, and those that we know will occur and can, to some degree, plan and prepare for. However, there is another group of changes which 'come to us', are brought to us, whether we like them or not, whether we are aware, or not. These are altogether more arbitrary and troublesome changes. Trying to ride a wave of change in the hope that we will somehow stay afloat and arrive at the shore is likely to become less and less attractive, given the complexity of the changes that we are passing through. Many people sat out the social changes of the 1960s and 1970s, waiting for the foamy turbulence to settle, relatively confident that the shoreline would look much as before. Almost everyone knows that the nature and the pace of social change is qualitatively different and this has an impact upon our work, social and personal lives. We are moving from one era into another. Whether the new era will usher in a time for renewed optimism and hope in human endeavour, or something altogether more deadly will, no doubt, hang in the balance for a long time to come, but it is happening. Existing frameworks of understanding are giving way. They no longer hold. They no longer offer convincing explanations or descriptions of the texture of our experience. New models can be only tentative, at best, for the time being. And yet, paradoxically, some realities remain much the same; some inescapable movements continue. Individual experience, however different and dislocated, is also connected to some familiar points: leaving school, becoming a citizen, taking up employment, establishing a relationship, and so on. It is the wider context against which our lives are lived that is undergoing upheaval, that is shifting so quickly.

New organisational problems

In organisations and institutions, so long under siege, or so it seems, the impact of the cumulative changes has begun to take effect at a new level. Accountability, deregulation, budgetary responsibility, and the shift of resources away from institutional solutions, have together contributed to the vital need to develop the capacity for strategic thinking and to increase our understanding of the similarities and differences between the processes of change, the phases of development and the experience of transformation. More than ever, those working in responsible positions in our organisations have to identify clearly where those organisations are, what are the characteristics of the 'reality of the situation' in which they are placed. In order to do that there is a need to look both inside and outside the organisation. Important issues are raised of choice and direction, dilemmas between competing priorities. The central purpose of the organisation has to be recast in the light of new realities. Although it is easy to recognise the need for reappraisal and change, as one manager did recently when he described the requirements of the situation he had uncovered for himself and his colleagues as requiring a 'change mode now' response, it is often more difficult to work out the implications or nature of that change.

Managing change

It is often only by attempting to implement a change, or living through a major upheaval, that we uncover all the resistances, difficulties and limitations we put in our own way, as a result of our fears and our limited understanding. There are few models of how change can come about elegantly and effectively, releasing the curiosity and creativity of those involved. We are more familiar with the discomfort of our frameworks being rendered useless, burnt up in front of our eyes. Often we simply do not know which questions to ask.

The context of events is moving fast, as the chapters in this book demonstrate. Restructuring the Health Service has been something of a political hobby from the 70's onwards. Many may not remember the

Salmon Report, the first of what became something of a torrent of reports that began to appear from the mid-1970s onwards. this was then swiftly followed by the Cumberlege and Griffiths reports in the 1980s – all before the reform of the Health Service that came at the end of the 1980s and into the 1990s. No organisation could expect to stand up to such a continuous assault upon its work and expect to continue to perform effectively. And yet what other response makes sense? – surely not to abandon all that one has held dear and simply drift along? How do we learn to manage ourselves through changes that no longer affect the structure, or the systems, the arrangements or the roles but the very nature of practice itself?

Under such circumstances 'managing' change is, perhaps, all that we can ever do. The idea that change can be made amenable to our direction, be brought under our 'control' and made to serve our purposes has to give way in the face of the present pace of change, whether social, economic, political or organisational: when change affects the very nature of practice itself, it becomes altogether more difficult to 'manage'. In such circumstances we are beginning to have to give up 'control' without surrendering our potential for influence. In some ways there has never been a greater opportunity for individuals to influence what is happening to them, but not by attempting to change the direction of events.

New and different forms of thinking will be required to work out where and how to manage individual contributions and, how to exercise influence. In less hierarchical structures, with greater accountability and yet tighter room for independent judgement, a paradox enters practice: how to act effectively and with a confident sense of judgement when your practice and that of others may not be in harmony?

- How do we learn to talk about differences without getting into 'rights' and 'wrongs', but into 'better' or 'less useful'?
- How do I learn to listen to your view and to understand it rather than feel judged or undermined because I view things differently?
- How many ways are there to do some things?
- How far does it matter that we differ?
- What do we do when someone else's practice is potentially unsafe and may threaten the reputation of us all?

These are not new matters in the workplace but they are more sharply present and they are more potentially disruptive than in the past. Under pressure, the opportunity to reflect and discuss issues of practice with a sense of calm and interest gives way to 'putting things right' (which can soon descend to 'covering things up'). Learning takes time and that is something we are all short of. So managing change at a personal level becomes one of the most essential attributes for any future practitioner. Self-management has to go along with a willingness to be accountable and the recognition that the complement to self-management is interdependence. Collaboration at a new level requires us to be engaged in more direct ways than have been necessary in the past. The potential for misdirection, getting lost, being overtaken by the immediate shifts and moves, and missing the deeper currents of events are all potential temptations of each phase of change. And if you are asking the wrong questions, any answers you get will not help you. If you do not know where you are going, wherever you end up will still only be somewhere else. Standing back may seem a luxury but travelling to nowhere is more than a pointless bus ride.

How we understand what is happening strongly influences what we decide to do. If we are using the wrong ideas, or have inadequate concepts, the actions that flow from them will not resolve our dilemma or further our development. However, having the right answer is of no use if we are unable to get people to make use of it, or if we are so crippled by doubt that we do not implement the actions that are required. Many of us hold ideas of change that are related to some (or perhaps all) of those outlined in Box 8.2. We often hold contradictory views of change within the space of the same conversation, depending upon which aspect of change is uppermost in our minds.

Box **8.2** Types of change

Incremental change   Changes are linear and accumulate in sequence.

Disruptive change   Change is an interruption to a predictable order or routine.

One-off change   Change is an interruption as a means of reorganisation, from one state to another.

Momentary change   There is a stable state to which we shall one day return.

Imposed change   External agents impose their ill-considered and unworkable ideas upon what is an already perfect system.

Interruptive change   Changes are deviations from an ordered and coherent system which is never allowed to operate because of such interruptions.

Revolutionary change   The political realities in the situation have changed and another group of people are now imposing their will upon what will take place. It is all out of our hands.

Random change   No one knows much about what is happening, so there is really no need to do any more than muddle on as before.

Programmed change   This is only a 'blip' on the graph of progress that underlies everything that goes on.

These kinds of views of change, while useful for many experiences or events, break down under turbulent and structural change that tears up the existing framework without replacing it with a new one immediately. Such change is akin to living through a revolution, and revolutions throughout history have usually cost lives. Whilst the context of change is revolutionary, individuals are still living their own lives with their own rhythms of change and development, their own experiences of life to accommodate to, and they are still making the journey from one stage or phase of their life to into another. Such transitions can make the challenge of external change even more difficult to work with. It can, of course, help too. Thinking about issues of transition, development and transformation are useful as ways of locating oneself in the personal picture, at the same time not forgetting the organisational one.

Transition

Transitions have elements of predictability, phases of activity, and thresholds that identify various stages along the route, whether it be the transition into a new position at work, a divorce, or into parenthood. The possibility of learning and integration are also important features of transitions, providing we understand that they have predictable and understandable phases from which lessons can be extracted.

Development

Development is often a process of qualitative change and is not necessarily gradual, or incremental. It is not necessarily related to travelling through a predictable transition. It can be experienced as a jump from one state of being to another. It is characterised by thresholds or frontiers and a strong conviction of a shift that is irrevocable. It is, however, linked to individual biography or 'lifescript', and is a living out of themes or issues at work in individual lives. The same features apply to organisational transformation. Development, then, is not random or unpredictable, however revolutionary it may appear to the subjects who are living through the change. For example, becoming a parent is a developmental shift (for most of us), just as taking on new responsibilities can be organisationally.

Transformation

Transformation is a 'qualitative shift of being', manifested in external and internal ways. It is a break with the past. It is the unpredicted shift to an altogether new level of operating. It is a move to a higher order of functioning which incorporates and integrates previous functions and will be manifested in changes in organisation, structure, function and process;

whilst identifiable through these differences and modifications, it is actually contained in none of them. Transformation is beyond singular manifestation and is apparent only as a result of appearing in all of them. (Whilst conversion experiences are obvious examples of a transformative change – not always for the good – there are other changes that take place at momentous points in a person's life that amount to a transformation. Perhaps the one most common and most turbulent is the crisis of mid-life, which often comes earlier in our present-day period of accelerated change.)

Working with change

All of us have to 'work with change' for or against, well or badly, through denial or even through a false acceptance. Many of us are quite happy to work with changes that we have striven for and desire to bring about. We are altogether less enamoured when the change is imposed and brought from outside. Working with change is not something that admits of a single solution: it requires effort and time, both of which, as we have already noted, are in short supply. It helps, however, to identify the number of events through which our lives are travelling and to distinguish them as externally imposed or internally inspired. A simple table may help (Table 8.1).

Whilst some events are easy to assign, others are open to various interpretations. For example, the end of a relationship may be a relief for one person (with costs nevertheless); for another it may be the heartbreaking end to a lifetime of commitment. Such personal meaning needs to be acknowledged and recognised. It is not what someone else regards for our proposals that is important, but what is significant for you, the reader. Events need to be placed where 'you' feel they are best placed. So, for some people, changes in the structure of their work will amount to a transfor-

Table 8.1 Imposed events; self-chosen events		
	External	**Internal**
Changes	Redundancy	Decision to change job
Transitions	Coping with illness	Move from parenting to children living away
Development phase	Redefining gender role	Mid-life changes
Transformation	Can't be 'me' any more	Downshifting*

*Term used to describe those who deliberately seek to reduce their financial and economic commitments, reduce their consumption habits and live a more modest and sustainable lifestyle.

mation that is generated from the outside whilst for others it will be no more than a change. For someone else, the importance of the transition from one role (practitioner to manager) will have greater weight than the changes to the structure within which they are working. For someone else, none of the changes taking place within the workplace will matter as much as managing a frail parent through the final stages of life. But all of us have a combination of external and internal experience that we are having to manage simultaneously.

Detecting change

The first sign of change is often one of unease: a suggestion that all is not well, that something has gone wrong, or is not working. Sometimes we know where the failure lies, but then it is usually someone else who should take action. Change and the responsibility for change lie outside us and we are free to blame or criticise. Only when we bring the change within our grasp, inside our own boundaries, can we move out of antagonism towards it, or righteous indignation about it. Only when we begin to ask: 'What else could there be?' or 'I'd like to see . . .' do we begin to form a productive relationship with what is happening. Only by forming a relationship toward what is happening can we begin to exert a useful influence. It is by developing a fascination, or a loving interest, that things begin to 'speak' back to us. Sometimes, when working with questions about change, the questions themselves come in search of us. Repeated reminders of a situation that demands attention appear time and time again, and we know that, sooner or later, we will have to put the time aside to respond. Some such changes stack up, just waiting for a glimpse of daylight to appear before us. They then fly out of the shadows and demand that we put off dealing with them no longer.

There are those changes, too, that we can barely look upon, because they bring us face to face with the 'shadow' of all we thought that we were about, where the 'darker side' of our motives becomes revealed and we have to face the pain of self-knowledge, acknowledge the hurt or the pain that we have, in part, inflicted. It is unpleasant and painful to have, at last, to acknowledge all that we have tried to put to one side or deny, but it pursues us until we recognise and work with it, or it helps to destroy us. Our freedom is related to the degree of intimacy we have developed with our own shadow. Sometimes it is the people coming towards us who bring with them the challenges and questions we next need to meet. Then we may have to look beyond the immediate needs of the situation, or what is being expressed, and ask: 'What are they seeking?', 'What more do they require of us?'. It may be straightforward and appropriate. It may not be within our power to offer, but always we will come to understand more about where we are, if we enquire into how they have come to find us and what it is they are in search of.

Some issues in managing change

The situation is hopeless but not serious. (Hungarian proverb)

The challenge of change is to remain effective, efficient and adaptable. Establishing realistic targets means having modest, achievable goals.

Choice is an aspect of the relationship we have with ourselves. It is not governed by external circumstances, although it is of course, influenced by them. The ability to see opportunities that exist before us and which may lead us forward distinguishes those who make something of change from those who are defeated by it. Unless we nurture and protect that inner space, where choice and development lie, we will be left responding mechanically, or we will drift aimlessly. We will become shaped by circumstances themselves, left without any firm resolve or clear sense of who we are.

RESPONSES TO CHANGE

When confronted with a challenging situation, most of us want to modify the situation to make it more amenable to our influence. We try hard to conceptualise and describe it in ways that make it easier for us to live with, or, if we have to change, to change in ways that seem most relevant to ourselves. This is often a way of changing the way we view our experience of what is happening to us, rather than changing what we do about it. Most of us would rather change our experience than risk changing our beliefs about what we might do about it. We have elaborate ways of changing in order not really to change but to convince ourselves that we are 'doing enough'. In other words, we are all good at pretending.

The maximum potential to have the greatest impact lies in sudden, unpredictable and disruptive, external intervention. It produces alarming confusion, rendering the subject open to large-scale manipulation, which takes a long time to settle. If this is done repeatedly, systems and individuals literally have 'no idea' of where they are and therefore have no considered response to offer.

Personal tasks in relation to change

Tasks	Skills
Enable the individual to take charge	Goal setting
Learn and manage the change process	Action planning
Manage consequences	Rehearsing
Monitor and evaluate results	Implementation
Bring action into the world	Homework and revision

Effective change comes about through choice

Before a change is attempted, the person, the situation and the world in which the person and situation exist must be sufficiently aligned for the person to manage what comes. The change may not be appreciable on the outside, but may represent a thorough internal revision of an individual's self-image. It may be making a statement to other people in the person's world which entails the need for some self-protection to manage and hold on to the changes they wish to implement. For some, the change will be experienced privately, an indication perhaps only to themselves of the gains they have made; for others, it is the social aspect of the change itself that marks the progress not only to themselves but to those around. The networks in which people live their lives get shaken, and some people may get left behind when a change takes place.

Personal problem solving is discussed later in this chapter. It is important to remember that nothing changes until we begin to act. It is not sufficient to have an insight or come to a decision for change to take place. Change has to be implemented. As the action stage approaches, we may well become nervous and anxious all over again at the prospect of what we now know we are committed to. We have to build a model for action that has manageable chunks of activity and realistic steps which we can, with a reasonable degree of confidence, expect to accomplish. Reviewing what actually happens in the light of experience is an additional and important source of further learning which makes the role of a speaking partner indispensable when wanting to deal with change effectively. A speaking partner is used to describe anyone who is in a helping relationship with the person undertaking the change, such as a personal development consultant, mentor, counsellor, therapist or peer. There is everything to learn from a success so that we can identify the skills and behaviours that can be drawn upon next time. Such exploration helps to generate positive behaviour and helps us move away from a remedial view of facing change.

There is no change without loss and no loss without change

Often we consider only one aspect of these two, interlinked and interdependent, forces of change and loss rather than both together, because one aspect is focused on at the expense of the other. For example, if I change my job, I am likely to focus upon the opportunities that lie ahead. If I am made redundant, I am all too likely to be aware of the loss that this represents. Helpful hints about the new opportunities that lie ahead are not likely to be welcomed. Those who are anxious about change are likely to anticipate the losses that will accompany any change and the temptation is to remain immobile for too long, finally finding some way to be pushed over the threshold at the last moment. On the other hand, those who cannot bear to wait for change to happen might well propel themselves into the future and, only once there, begin to face the loss of what has been left behind. Either way, both have to be managed and dealt with, the loss and the change – the shedding of what has been left behind and the taking on of what we find in the new situation awaiting us.

TYPES OF CHANGE

It is useful to consider the types of change we experience as falling into four main groups:

1. Changes that are sought voluntarily, such as going on holiday or choosing to get married.
2. Events that happen involuntarily, whether we want them to or not – events over which we have no choice, such as becoming retired or being made redundant.
3. Events that we know will happen and that we can plan for, events which are predictable.
4. Events that affect us without any forewarning and are unpredictable, such as accidents.

There are, of course, inter-relationships between the groups, as shown in the examples given in Table 8.2.

Some changes are to be expected, given the culture and times in which we live. Other changes are much more idiosyncratic, or at odds with what else is happening to people like ourselves. This can create difficulties for us adjusting and understanding what has happened. Our individual biography, or life script, will have a crucial influence upon what happens to us and the way in which we respond. However, many people adopt an attitude to life which ensures that much of what happens to them is experienced as being involuntary and unpredictable. They take little initiative in finding out what is likely to happen and face change only when it is forced upon them. The more we take such a passive attitude, the more we are likely to feel we have little significant influence over our lives. Part of the helping process is to enable the individual to develop an increasing awareness and therefore

Table 8.2 Examples of possible inter-relationships between different types of events

	Voluntary	Involuntary
Predictable	Applying for promotion Marriage Having children	Retirement Being 'moved' in an organisation
Unpredictable	Surprise party Sudden holiday	Accident Relocation

more capacity to take charge of what happens to them, and to become an 'actor' in their lives rather than to feel a 'pawn'.

Traumatic change is usually experienced as involuntary and unpredictable.

MANAGING CHANGE

There is an old Sufi story of Nasrudin who had lost his keys in the dark and was fumbling around attempting to find them. His friend approached him and asked what he was doing. Nasrudin stopped and looked up at his friend and explained that he was looking for his keys under the light of the streetlamp. 'Where,' the friend asked, 'did you lose your keys?' 'Over there,' said Nasrudin, pointing some way off into the inky blackness. 'But it is no good looking over there, because it is too dark to see anything. At least there is enough light here to see what I am doing!'.

There are many factors that influence how each of us will approach change, the beliefs we hold about change, our relationship with change and our capacity for implementing change. Knowledge and understanding of these factors are important for a helper. The following section highlights these factors and also gives strategies that will be useful to the helper.

Factors that affect the management of change include:

- the context of the change
- the frame of reference we have for this experience
- the weight of the particular event itself
- what else is going on in our world
- how far this change is related to the life stage of the individual
- the extent to which the individual has a zone of stability in their personal life (If work is changing, how stable is the pattern of personal relationships, for example, as a way of compensating?)
- the emotional stress of the event and the strain of the process
- the cognitive readjustment necessary to make sense of the process.

The need for our experience to make sense is a vital element in what makes the change process so ambivalent and uncertain. Even changes we wish for bring a disturbance to our world view and sense of how things are. This makes individuals vulnerable for a period.

Helping strategies include:

- filtering experiences and reducing the workload
- queuing: listing things in priority order to give ourselves more flexibility and fewer demands
- reducing our usual standards of performance, where possible, to an 'OK enough' standard, as a way of freeing up energy to manage the change itself

- withdrawal: taking time out, as long as we realise that we will have to return to the situation, can sometimes be useful. Withdrawal has both positive and negative aspects, when, for example, it leads to failure of nerve to return to deal with the situation.

PERSONAL PROBLEM SOLVING

People in the helping professions often refer to the difficulties of those seeking help as having 'personal problems' in a loose kind of way, well aware that not all the difficulties people experience are either 'personal', in the sense that they have their origin in decisions individuals have made for themselves, or 'problems', in the sense that their dilemmas have a clear cause let alone solution. In what sense is the loss of a parent a problem? Rather, it is a naturally occurring life crisis which the majority of people will have to face one day. Some people will meet this and other crises with little or no need of outside support; others will not. This is not a judgement upon those who, at times of crisis, seek out a listening ear to help them shape their experience into understanding. Some people are fortunate to live in a network of support that is freely available, but many people have no such network. In times of difficulty they are without close contacts to share their difficulties and must look outside for support. It is often the case that people who are seeking help find it difficult to make the request openly and may offer a more tangible and practical need as the reason for seeking help in the beginning. In this way we may adopt a heroic attitude to what we face, struggle on bravely (or so we think) and end up with a much bigger crisis of stacked-up unfinished, and often unacknowledged, issues awaiting – all at the time when our system is at its most compromised from our efforts at putting things off for so long. We need to be alert to clues that might suggest the presence of other issues or concerns.

Uncertainty

When someone says they 'don't know what to do', they are really saying that they have no reference system for making a choice. They do not have a secure enough base upon which to make a selection. A reference system for making decisions about whether to stay in a relationship, whether to buy a new house, or to change your job, will not necessarily be the same. However, most people use the same strategy to make almost all their decisions, or they try to (they usually describe this as being 'consistent', something that 'life' itself is not, so why should they be?). This means they will be good at deciding some things (things that are related to the kind of activity that the strategy was designed to deal with) and not others. They are unlikely to know why this is so, or even to realise that there are a range of activities or decisions for which the strategy serves them well, since the development of such a strategy is largely unconscious and related to underlying beliefs. They will then use the same strategy over and over again, until it works. This is a sure way of perpetuating failure: if the strategy did not work the first time, then it won't on the fifty-third occasion either. If at first you don't succeed, then do something else. If, for example, you use pictures from your past to determine what you do in the future, you are likely to condemn yourself to living out the same kinds of relationships and to make the same kinds of choices you have made before. You may then be doing little but repeating the past in slightly different versions. Such a strategy can be useful for solving conceptual problems and planning things, but it is not a useful way of solving 'people' problems, especially if you don't want to end up in the same place again.

When people confess to not knowing what to do in a particular situation, it is not that they lack the kind of information they need, despite what they might say. Usually, they have more information than they could ever hope to need. Most people interested in dieting, for example, know more about diets and calories than they need to, to lose weight. Such information is not crucial to solving their problem. What they lack is not information, but a way of knowing how to evaluate it usefully in relation to the outcome they are seeking.

The importance of context

All problems occur within some context. The context is determined by what the individual decides to pay attention to and what is 'screened out', and what people pay attention to is determined by what they value. When people do not know what to do, they do not know what to value. Meaning lies in people, and people code their experiences differently. We may all experience the same event, but each of us will represent it differently in unique internal patterns. There is a tremendous difference between an experience and how it is represented, very much like the difference between the meal and the menu. Most of the time, people are responding not to what is actually 'out there' in the world, but to what they think it might mean, what it 'should' mean, or what they believe they 'ought' to do about it. They continually look for what is the same in this experience compared with the past and not for what is novel and different.

However, effective decision making is about choice. To have only one option is to be no more than a robot; two alternatives equals a dilemma and is like operating with an on/off switch. Only when you have at least three possibilities does choice begin. One way of defining choice is as a 'multiple response to the same stimulus'. For most of us, most of the time, choice is about having a range of ways to go after what we want. Choice is related to outcome.

Outcome

When making a choice it is therefore important to know clearly and unambiguously what it is you want, the outcome you are aiming to achieve. This needs to be stated accurately and specifically, because sloppy language produces sloppy results. The 'best person for the job' can bring you a lot of surprises, if 'best' is not defined any more carefully than that. Once you have a clear outcome, you have to have the behavioural resources to gain it. This requires behavioural flexibility, which is often limited by underlying beliefs and concerns that are not always known consciously.

Most personal problems have some function or purpose in the total life circumstances of that individual. Somehow and at some time it made sense to acquire whatever habit or behavioural pattern the person now seeks to change. If change were such a simple and straightforward matter, helpers would quickly be out of business. The fact is that problems give people certain kinds of secondary rewards – ways of getting certain kinds of attention that are extremely important to them and which they believe they cannot get in other ways. If, for example, I complain repeatedly of my ill-health and this gets me noticed, I may remain heavily invested in staying the way I am, despite my complaints, since this gets me something I want: time, sympathy and attention. Making technical suggestions to solve a personal problem is the least difficult aspect of helping someone to change. It is more important to establish what the pay-off of the problem is and to find ways for the client to obtain the same reward more safely and more effectively.

Assumptions

A variety of approaches have been designed to help individuals solve personal problems. Many are recent in origin and derive from techniques developed in the 'new therapies'. The approach outlined here is based on a learning and information model. The underlying assumptions are:

- People can learn to solve their own problems and, when they do, they acquire skills transferable to other situations.
- Many people lack sufficient information in their awareness to solve their problems. The role of the helper is to help them to raise the information into their awareness so they can act for themselves.
- Many problems are capable of improvement through the help of another.

Such an approach would not be suitable for dealing with long-standing emotional difficulties or critically serious disruptions to an individual's life, unless it were accompanied by skilled specialist help. It is important, therefore, for anyone undertaking the role of helper to ask themselves whether they possess the necessary skills to help and whether this approach is suitable for the problem. Force-field analysis is a further resource for personal problem solving and draws on the work of Kurt Lewin and Gerard Egan.

PROBLEM SOLVING AND DECISION MAKING

It may be unfortunate, but it is true, that the only behaviour you can do something about is your own. You cannot change other people, you can only help them to change if they want to. The problem may appear to be centred in someone else, but the only parts you can act upon immediately are those that influence and affect you. Once you have taken the first step and have begun to concentrate on your own behaviour, you can begin to apply the steps shown in Box 8.3.

Box 8.3 Steps to take in problem solving

1. Identify the problem Express the essence of the problem in a simple sentence that a 7-year-old child would understand. Keep at this stage until you get it. This may mean facing there is not one problem, but several, all wrapped up in a situation. Then you have to decide which 'bit' you are going to tackle first.

2. What have you done so far? Briefly outline the strategies attempted and the results obtained so far. Explore when and how you first became aware of the issue and the signals that indicated it was an issue. What are the signals 'now' which indicate that the problem is about to appear? (This is about finding out what the lead-up to the problem is.)

3. What have you not done but could attempt? Explore alternative options and ask yourself, non-judgementally, why they have not been attempted or, if they have, what happened? This is to begin identifying the underlying restrictions of belief.

4. What gets in the way? What are the factors that might be holding you back? What might you be saying to yourself that limits you? What other self-imposed limitations might there be that you might need to explore? (Reference to personal myths may help.)

5. What do you want? What outcome is sought in solving this problem? Keep on going with this until you have a positive and specific description that you are clear is potentially achievable. It has to be capable of achievement by you and, once achieved, sustained by you.

Box 8.3 Cont'd

6. Is it realistic? How does this outcome stand up to rigorous analysis in the light of potential experience? Modify the plan and do more work, rather than go out and discover more pain and frustration.

7. Reduce it to manageable chunks Break down the overall aim to manageable, time-related pieces. Make sure the time scale is realistic.

8. Implementation Decide when the first steps will be put into effect. Ensure there is sufficient support, if needed. Consider what will happen if the unexpected appears and confounds your efforts.

9. Evaluate Review the actual events against your expectations. Invite feedback.

A mnemonic for problem solving

This is a way of thinking that is useful; one that can be operated anywhere and for almost any problem:

P   Pose the problem accurately.
R   Refine the problem areas into manageable chunks.
O   Outline the 'right' kind of questions to ask.
B   Bring back the data – information that is accurate and relevant to the problem.
L   Look for solutions.
E   Evaluate options.
M   Make a decision.
S   So what next?

The three components

To solve any problem successfully, you require as much reliable information as you can get. There are three aspects to the solution of any problem. There is a knowing component, a feeling component, and an action component. Most of the time it is much easier to gather the information than it is to act upon it, and the way a person feels about things will have great influence upon what they decide to do.

Knowing

To gain information quickly, it is often better to seek someone who already knows the information you require than to try to do it all by yourself. But make sure the source of the information you seek is reliable. It is your responsibility to ensure that the information is accurate and relevant to your needs. Ask yourself:

1. What do I already know about the problem?
2. What do I need to know?
3. How could I find out?
4. Who might be able to help?

Feeling

Having information relating to a problem does not always lead to an individual taking positive action. The evidence connecting cigarette smoking and lung cancer is not sufficient in itself to stop many people from smoking, although it probably makes most people think harder about giving it up or to feel guilty if they continue. For some people, to admit that they have a particular problem would be to lose self-respect or self-esteem. Denying the problem is a way of avoiding having to confront the implications and the challenge to an individual's self-image. Alcoholics often refuse to admit they have a 'drink' problem until it is acute and therefore harder to change. Sometimes solving a problem is resisted or avoided because the person concerned would then have to consider what to do instead of complaining or feeling sorry for themselves. Ask yourself:

1. How do I feel about the problem?
2. Do I feel that way at other times?
3. How important is it to me to solve the problem?
4. What effect would it have upon my life if I were without it?

Acting

Knowing all that is required to solve a problem and then becoming motivated merely gets one to the starting point. A problem is solved only by doing something about it. It is important to identify the sequence of activities and skills required to achieve a solution, and to isolate those that are most difficult or that require most support or practice before they are tried out. Once the behaviours that are most difficult or risky have been identified, they can be practised away from the situation until confidence has been developed and the person feels easier about trying them out in the real situation. Talking is a form of practice, and so is role play. The advantage of this kind of practice is that it provides an opportunity to evaluate the results in a risk-free environment, so that anything with which the person is not satisfied can be modified.

Reviewing

Stay involved. Once you have put a plan into action, it is important to check how you went about it so that you can remember it the next time or go over the areas of difficulty. Review enables people to build on their success and to identify skills they already have and use.

REFERENCES

Edelwich, J. & Brodsky, A. (1980). *Burn-Out: Stages of Disillusionment in the Helping Professions.* New York: Human Sciences.

Further Reading

Bolles, R.N. (1981). *The Three Boxes of Life and How to Get Out of Them.* Berkeley: Ten Speed Press.

Schon, D. (1987). *Educating the Reflective Practitioner.* San Francisco: Jossey Bass.

Schutz, W. (1984). *The Truth Option.* Berkeley: Ten Speed Press.

Taylor, B. (1996). *Helping People Change.* Boston Spa: Oasis Publications.

Taylor, B. (1997). *Where Do I Go From Here?* Boston Spa: Oasis Publications.

Taylor, B. (1998). *Working With Others,* 5th edn. Boston Spa: Oasis Publications.

Organisational change

Stephanie Carson

KEY ISSUES

◆ Description of different organisational cultures and structures

◆ Models for change

◆ How evidence-based practice can be incorporated into business planning and performance management

◆ Examples of evidence-based practice in decision making by commissioners

◆ Outline of features of successful organisations

◆ Framework (questions) for you to identify your own organisational structure and culture

INTRODUCTION

This chapter gives the organisational context for evidence-based practice and how it may be used as a driver to change service provision. Healthcare services exist in a constantly changing environment. Technological advances are being made all the time which push the barriers of medicine forward and bring yet further change. It is important that you as a practitioner understand the relationship between organisational structure, culture and strategy, so that you can understand and influence the decision-making process.

Conventional descriptions of organisational cultures and structures are outlined, so that you can begin to identify the key features of your own organisation. An overview of the business planning process is given, from the perspective of the Trust or Provider organisation. The ways that evidence-based practice can be incorporated within planning are suggested for your consideration. Evidence-based practice is now becoming an increasingly accepted indicator on which commissioning decisions at health authority level are being made, as well as commissioning within a primary care framework. These changes present the practitioner with exciting opportunities to influence which services are commissioned, and how those services are provided.

A series of questions for you to ask yourself about your own organisation will help you identify the particular culture and style, in order to explore the possibilities of using evidence-based practice within a change management framework.

ORGANISATIONAL CULTURE

Management literature abounds with definitions of organisational culture, but the simplest which encompasses the essentials has been distilled from Schein (1985): 'the way organisational members behave and the values that are important to them'. Put even more simply this can be stated as 'The way we do things around here'. Within this section, the main features of some of the most frequently used models of organisational culture are highlighted.

Mechanistic versus organic

The mechanistic organisation is characterised by centralised decision-making processes. Rules and procedures abound and structures tend to be extremely hierarchical. In a mechanistic culture, communication is more likely to be vertical (i.e. top down) and to a lesser extent bottom up. This reflects the structure of vertical units or divisions.

Conversely, organic cultures are very flexible, decision making is decentralised and there are few rules or procedures. Communication can be more easily facilitated laterally (i.e. across the organisation) and matrix working (described in more detail under Organisational structures) is more likely to develop.

Role versus task

This is similar to the above dichotomy, so that the role culture tends towards bureaucracy and hierarchy. The culture is secure and predictable, and seen to be protected by the rules and procedures. Individuals' roles and responsibilities and positions of authority are regarded as important (i.e. position power), the *who* (their roles and responsibilities) being the focal point.

Task-oriented cultures concentrate on the *what*, being project or job oriented. These are flexible and fully integrated organisations which can respond quickly and creatively.

Club

The club model is common within healthcare organisations, particularly within the medical profession or dentistry, but it also exists within other professional groups. This is about personal power. The individual is entrepreneurial, and the organisation provides the administrative resources. This can lead to tensions in the system such as the professional versus corporate approach. This has been true in the past within National Health Service (NHS) Trusts on issues such as drug therapies or operating costs, and reinforces the need to base both professional and managerial decisions on evidence-based practice where possible.

Learning

The learning culture tends to be fostered by organisations that are flexible, open and pragmatic. A culture of enquiry develops together with autonomy, creativity and entrepreneurship amongst employees.

The culture of the organisation depends to a large extent on the main function of the organisation. For example, the organic – task culture is more suited to the needs of the marketing environment. In healthcare services many of the rules and procedures are there to protect the individuals receiving treatment. Similarly, while clinical autonomy is to be encouraged, too much creativity amongst surgeons when operating may not foster confidence.

You can already begin to see how the different cultures will react to, hinder or drive changes. This becomes more obvious when we look at the structure of the organisation and link this with the organisational culture in the next section.

Reflection   Four descriptions of possible organisational cultures are given: Mechanistic versus Organic, Role versus Task, Club, and Learning. Which aspects most closely resemble your understanding of the culture in which you work?

ORGANISATIONAL STRUCTURES

In this section we look at different types of structures within healthcare organisations and how these link with the cultures described above. The principal advantages and disadvantages of each are listed and it is important to remember that these structures are changing and evolving as the organisation grows and develops.

Centralisation versus decentralisation

Within centralised structures senior managers keep control over making and taking most decisions. Employees lower down the structure may have the authority to implement the decisions, once the process of implementation has been identified by senior managers (i.e. the *what, how and when*).

In decentralised structures senior managers will tend to encourage development of decision making to the lowest appropriate level possible within the structure (i.e. *who*). Advantages and disadvantages of centralised and decentralised structures are shown in Table 9.1.

There are four main structures common within healthcare organisations, with variations on a theme based around these as organisations evolve. We have also added a fifth, as applied to the concept of shared governance. Examples of healthcare structures based on service providers within the NHS are given below.

Table 9.1 Advantages and disadvantages of centralised and decentralised structures

	Advantages	Disadvantages
Centralisation	Consistency of approach Easier to coordinate Easier to implement and control change	Less flexibility Slow response to change Tends to be bureaucratic Overspecialisation can occur Lack of coordination
Decentralisation	More flexible Encourages innovation and creativity Greater ownership and improved motivation of staff	Difficulties in coordination if strategic goals unclear Problems in linking autonomy with responsibility and accountability

Functional structure

This is a common structure within NHS Trusts, working on a directorate basis (see Fig. 9.1). The structure is based on the specialist tasks to be carried out and is centralised. This structure can be easily controlled by a chief executive or board, who can also maintain a strategic awareness. It can be a very efficient structure, which allows managers to develop specialist expertise.

Disadvantages include possible difficulties in succession planning, organisational flexibility and potential internal rivalry (medical versus surgical?).

Divisional structure

This is a decentralised structure and another common model for NHS organisations (see Fig. 9.2). These organisations are more readily able to

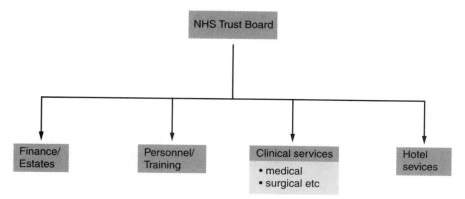

Figure 9.1 Functional structure (e.g. National Health Service Trust).

adapt to change, being more responsive than the above model. There are also opportunities for general as well as specialist managers, who can then be entrepreneurial if desired.

Drawbacks include potential duplication of effort and conflicts for resources. There may also be problems coordinating the different divisions and agreeing internal costs.

Entrepreneurial structure

This structure reflects some of the general practitioner fundholding practices in the early stages of their development (see Fig. 9.3). Primary care

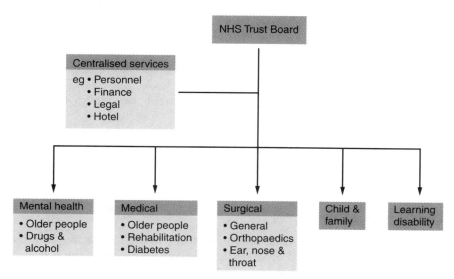

Figure 9.2 Divisional structure (e.g. National Health Service Trust).

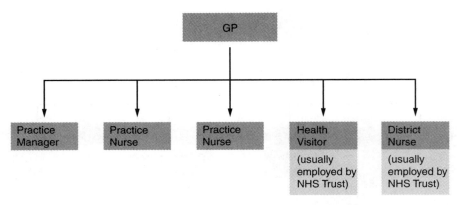

Figure 9.3 Entrepreneurial structure (e.g. general practitioner fundholding practice).

organisations are a good example of how dynamic the structures can be to reflect the needs of the organisation at the time. There is little or no division of responsibility (at a strategic rather than clinical level). This allows the key developer to regulate its growth in the initial stages, but can also be hampered by the individual's lack of specialist knowledge in key areas. This model does not operate as well once mergers or practice consortia develop, creating a more complex organisation.

Matrix structure

This is another example of a decentralised structure and may be partially applied within NHS Trusts on a temporary project team basis, or within a locality model (see Fig. 9.4). The driver for this model is the need to provide services on a geographical or 'patch' basis. The advantages of this structure are that decisions can be made at a local level based on the local population's healthcare needs. It makes optimum use of the organisation's skills and resources, and reduces bureaucracy. It also allows easier access to other agencies such as social services to provide an integrated health and social care package.

Potential problems are caused by the difficulties in implementation, high overhead costs and the time taken for the decision-making process to be completed. It can also be difficult to work out on a day-to-day basis just who you are accountable to and for what.

Shared governance

A more recent approach introduced from work in the USA advocated by Tim Porter O'Grady is that of shared governance. This structure is based on the principle that in order to effect change you must begin with the

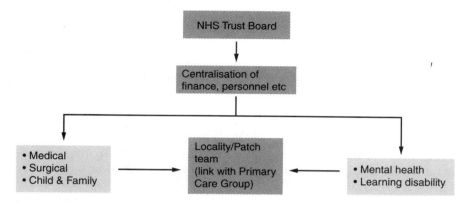

Figure 9.4 Matrix structure (e.g. locality model).

largest group that is closest to the point of service. In healthcare, this is obviously nursing. In some healthcare organisations shared governance is now implemented across all disciplines. The system reflects a clinical rather than administrative base. Decision making is decentralised, accountability is at the level of the individual and therefore horizontal lines of communication are developed. There are four underlying principles:

1. partnership at all levels
2. accountability in every role
3. equity between participants
4. ownership and investment by all.

There are variations which can be adapted from O'Grady's original models (Porter O'Grady 1995), but all include clinical accountabilities for practice, research, education and quality. You can begin to see from this brief outline that this approach links well into evidence-based practice and clinical governance (see also Chapter 10). Once the structure is in place, there are four levels of decision making:

1. collecting data
2. collecting data and making recommendations
3. collecting data and making recommendations and acting upon these
4. 'do as I do'.

The four principles of partnership, accountability, equity and ownership – investment echo the themes running throughout current healthcare and social policy.

Key points

• Four models of organisational structure have been described: functional, divisional, entrepreneurial and matrix.

- Shared governance is based on a horizontal system design and links into the concept of clinical governance.
- Which structure is the basis for the model within your organisation?
- Are there examples of other substructures within the organisation? If so, how might these help or hinder change and the use of evidence-based practice?

MODELS OF ORGANISATIONAL CHANGE

Whichever of the above cultures and structures you work in, the one constant will be change: a change in the remit of the organisation, a merger or takeover (especially within the NHS). There are three principal models of managing change, which lend themselves to incorporating evidence-based practice to differing degrees. Any change can be an opportunity as well as a threat. In learning about these models and understanding the change process, you can see why these changes occur and how you may be able to influence the outcomes in relation to changes in the provision of healthcare services and, importantly, improve these services for the individuals receiving the care.

Action research model

This model is also referred to as action learning, and is probably the most useful of the models described in this section in relation to evidence-based practice in healthcare. A definition put forward by French and Bell (1984, pp. 98–99), states:

> *Action Research is research on action with the goal of making that action more effective. Action refers to programmes and interventions designed to solve a problem or improve a condition . . . action research is the process of systematically collecting data about an ongoing system relative to some objective, goal, or need of that system; taking action by altering selected variables within the system based both on the data and on hypotheses; and evaluating the results of actions by collecting more data.*

Usually a small group is formed, comprising:

- an organisational representative(s) (i.e. senior manager(s))
- the subject (i.e. the service or location where the change will be occurring)
- a change agent, who may be internal or external to the organisation.

An iterative process then begins, starting with data collection. Hypotheses are then formulated from the above participants, an action plan is identified, implemented and finally evaluated.

Evidence-based practice may be crucial to this approach, firstly in identifying the range of solutions and secondly in assessing and choosing the one that is most appropriate.

The possible difficulties with this model arise from the reliance on compliance with all parties concerned and not solely senior management. The feeling of the need to change within the relevant part of the organisation is also central to the process. This will not, however, always lessen individual and personal anxieties about the impact of the proposed change. These effects and their impact should not be underestimated when you come to implement your action plan.

Three-step model of change

In this model the 'felt need' is again important to any change taking place. To ensure that any change is established on a longer-term basis, this model looks first at jettisoning existing ways of functioning and then moves to the new approach. This is referred to as unfreezing–moving–refreezing. Ways of unfreezing (similar to the action research model stage of research) can involve familiar processes such as team building, where the issues are analysed and problems identified to prove to all parties that there is a need for change. The stage of moving may require a new organisational structure and processes to achieve changes in behaviours, beliefs and values that are long lasting and do not allow a gradual slip back into the old familiar ways of doing things. This striving for a more permanent change in behaviours underpins this approach and aims to bypass the 'latest fad' in management techniques reaction to change. This is particularly important in healthcare where change is an ever-present feature owing to technological advances, research, policy and economic influences. Note as well that these models are iterative or cyclical in nature.

The final phase of the process is the refreezing, which will maintain the new balance within the organisation. This is reinforced by new policies and practices and is again a crucial stage for the utilisation of evidence-based practice and maintaining changes brought about by its introduction to an area of clinical work.

Phases of planned change

There are many models that have elaborated on the above three phases, with up to eight different steps outlined in detail. For the purposes of this chapter, we will remain with a four-step model (see Box 9.1) which highlights the essential stages of the process of change.

This model, described by Bullock and Batten (1985) looks at change phases and change processes. The phases are separate states which the organisation migrates through as it addresses the planned changes. The processes are the methods by which the changes are made in moving the organisation from one phase to another.

Box 9.1 Four-step model of the essential stages of the change process

1. Exploration phase In this initial stage, the organisation decides whether it wishes to make the change or stay with the 'do nothing' option. Once the decision has been taken to make changes, the resources required to plan the changes are identified. Often external assistance such as a facilitator is brought in to aid the process. A specification is agreed so that each party is clear about the remit and expectations of the changes about to take place.

2. Planning phase As with the earlier two models, an information-gathering exercise then takes place to identify the key issues of the problem and agree the change goals. The action plan to achieve these goals is then drawn up and agreed by the senior management.

3. Action phase This stage is about gaining general support and agreement within the organisation and implementing the changes outlined in the action plan. Evaluation is an important part of this process so that necessary adjustments can be made.

4. Integration phase This is a period of consolidation and stability following the changes to ensure they become embedded within the organisation's operations and are not simply overlaid on top of existing arrangements. Training appropriate personnel is usually a crucial process, and again an area that lends itself to incorporating the evidence-based practice which may have triggered the process initially.

Key points

- Models of change all share at least three basic elements: recognition of the need to change (situational analysis), implementation of an action plan for change, followed by a period of consolidation and evaluation.

INCORPORATING EVIDENCE-BASED PRACTICE INTO THE BUSINESS PLANNING AND PERFORMANCE MANAGEMENT FRAMEWORK

Evidence-based practice planning

Within the healthcare sector there has been gradually increasing pressure to ensure greater accountability, not only from a management perspective, but also for practitioners. Evidence-based practice is a useful tool to develop and increase awareness of its benefits to a wider group of stakeholders. In the private sector, financial factors have been the main driver for improved effectiveness and efficiency, and this is where many of the performance indicators within healthcare services originated.

Initially there was a concentration on inputs as an indicator to service quality. More recently, the importance of the processes was recognised, but again only telling part of the story. Regardless of the approach to quality (and it is not the remit of this chapter to reopen that interesting debate), the whole picture needs to be considered (i.e. inputs, process and outcomes). Evidence-based practice provides proven methods of approaches to patient care, giving details of the required inputs (resources), the process or treatment and the expected outcomes. It is therefore of potential benefit to all parties. Many existing performance indicators look at an area in isolation and the information can be interpreted in a variety of interesting ways. A prime example of this is length of stay for inpatients and finished consultant episodes (FCEs), neither of which reflect the type of care or the quality of care received by an individual.

The business planning process is crucial to developing the organisation's direction, and the business plan falls out of the strategic plan. It is possible that some of you reading this chapter feel that you have little, if any, influence on the strategic plans of your organisation. It is important to appreciate the lines of communication within the organisation (think about the structure here) and to identify management and others who under-stand the principles of evidence-based practice.

It is also essential to spend some time discovering what other examples of evidence-based practice there are within the organisation and how these were introduced. In the NHS the concept of clinical governance very clearly underlines the accountability issue and creates an excellent opportunity for broaching the introduction of specific examples of evidence-based practice.

You obviously need to be clear about the message you are trying to put over and that you have the relevant articles to hand: earlier chapters outline how to approach this aspect. However, clinical audit has been encouraged for several years within the NHS and there will be examples of good practice following audit projects within your own organisation.

You can put the message across in a language that managers will follow easily, avoiding too much medical or professional jargon in the initial stages. It is usually best received in the corporate context of benefits to individuals receiving improved care, more effective care, better use of existing resources, etc. This can be done as part of the business planning process and throughout the year, developing business cases as necessary.

To start on the process, if it is the first time that you have done this, or if you are familiar with the method but find you become bogged down in detail and lose sight of the overall objectives, there are useful techniques that you can try. These are even more helpful in simply getting started when you have lots of ideas, but cannot form them into a cohesive whole:

1. **Relationship diagram** The words in a relationship diagram show the differing factors and the lines show potential links or relationships between them. You may need to draw more than one diagram if the ideas start flowing thick and fast. Figure 9.5 shows an early thought processes for this chapter.

2. **Rich picture** This technique is taken from the Checkland soft systems analysis (Checkland 1981) and can also prove to be a useful starting point. It should be stressed that these diagrams are usually working diagrams for the author and not generally for public viewing, unless there are specific reasons for wishing to demonstrate the developmental stages. Figure 9.6 below again shows an early version of a rich picture for this chapter. In some cases only drawings are used with no supplementary wording involved. Flip chart paper is the best size, so that you have plenty of space to keep enlarging the picture as you go.

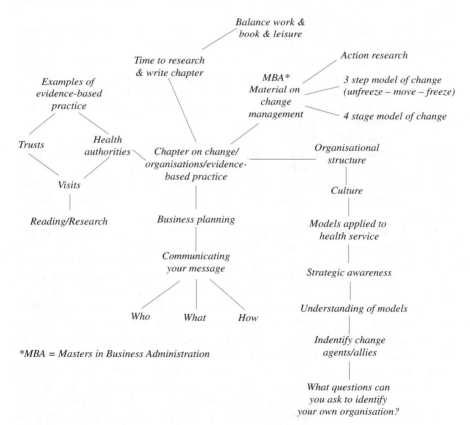

Figure 9.5 Relationship diagram for developing this chapter.

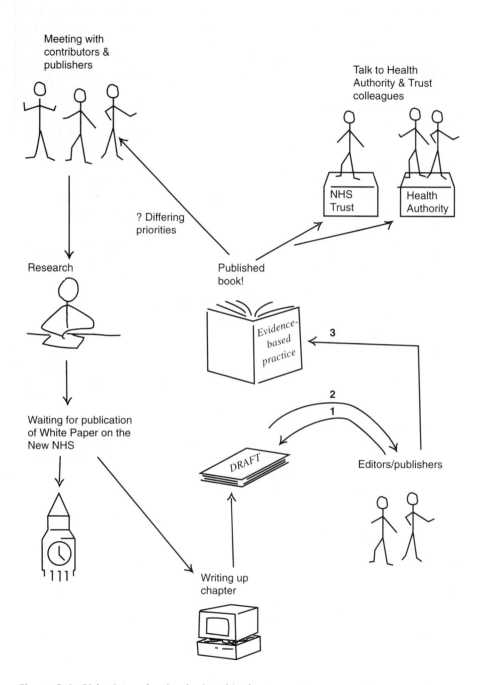

Figure 9.6 Rich picture for developing this chapter.

The business planning cycle links into the financial year from 1 April to 31 March, and in many organisations the process starts the previous August or September. Individual departments or divisions can produce their own detailed business plan, which can then be distilled and incorporated into the main organisational plan or summary. In aiming to gain some recognition, you need to look at how evidence-based practice links into national healthcare policies and whether there are any regional or local initiatives that will provide an opening. A good starting point is always to have a look at the latest *Priorities and Planning Guidance,* which can be obtained directly from the NHS Executive. Health Service Circulars (HSCs) containing the latest guidance are always circulated to NHS Trust and health authority chief executives. For anyone working in these organisations, it may be more cost effective and quicker to acquire a copy from either the chief executive's office or the human resource/ personnel department.

Remember, the first step is about getting other people to listen to or read about your ideas for improving care. When writing a business plan, look at other examples, not just from your own organisation, but others for a different perspective. Writing in the corporate style of your own organisation is important: people are more likely to read information which is in a familiar style. For example, if the plan is in tabular format, then avoid writing pages of text that will sit on a senior manager's desk unread.

Pathways of care provide an example of identifying the processes involved in particular types of care. In some cases, the predicted outcomes are also included within the pathway. The most common pathways developed by NHS Trusts are usually based on surgical procedures such as fractured neck of femur, mainly because these represent discrete episodes of care. Asthma pathways across both acute and primary care services are being developed and in some Trusts stroke pathways have been produced. Much has already been written about developing pathways and how this can link into the audit cycle. Suffice it to say here that, if you build in expected outcomes and base the pathway on evidence-based practice you are well on the way to improving healthcare.

So far we have talked about evidence-based practice as if it exists for all aspects of healthcare. There are obviously many areas for which no evidence is yet available – in some areas, it may always prove difficult to produce evidence. This situation opens up yet more possibilities:

- the development of multiprofessional projects or research (as discussed in previous chapters)
- the ability to produce reasoned arguments as to why a particular type of intervention should take place (in some cases the probable impact of not intervening and the long-term consequences). This is not to encourage any professional 'preciousness', which would severely undermine the good work of earlier stages.

The importance of including reference to evidence-based practice within a business plan or more detailed business case is crucial. It will facilitate the organisation's role within the commissioning framework. Health authorities now use evidence-based practice as a tool to inform their commissioning strategy. It is not the only aspect that they consider, but it is certainly discussed in key areas. Some well-known examples are shown in Box 9.2.

A note of caution is necessary here: health authorities have to undertake a difficult balancing act between providing healthcare for the many, specialised healthcare for the few, and limited resources for both. Some of the results of commissioning decisions may mean that you as practitioners have to change your approach to some interventions, or the interventions being prioritised lower down the scale than you may feel is comfortable. Ask yourself why this discomfort is there: is it on behalf of the individual you are helping or have helped, or is it the change and perceived threat to your professional skills?

Implementation of evidence-based practice: theory into practice

Assuming that your bid has been successful and you are now at the implementation stage, or that your idea required no additional resources and senior managers have jumped at the opportunity, you now need to implement the scheme. In changing practice it is essential to identify all the stakeholders (include the representatives of those who will be receiving the changed intervention where possible) and to communicate the changes

---

Box 9.2 Examples of the use of evidence-based practice in commissioning strategy

Glue ear or otitis media   Studies have shown that, rather than operating on so many children as a matter of course, for a significant number of children an operation is unnecessary, the infection having resolved (i.e. dry taps – no glue ear at the time of surgery). This is not to say that no children would benefit from surgical intervention, but that a change in practice can identify those requiring surgery and prevent children from receiving anaesthetic for no reason.

Asthma   The use of asthma metered-dose inhalers has been shown to be more effective when the additional Volumatic spacer devices are used. Not only is there improved effectiveness, but also improved quality and a decrease in associated costs.

proposed. The style of communication has to be thought through carefully in the same way as presenting the message to senior managers. The mode of communication may also be different. You would not use the same language to relatives or voluntary groups as you would when explaining to colleagues. This may appear to be common sense, but when carried away in the middle of detail it can be easily overlooked.

There may also be groups that you need to involve in the earlier listening and analysis stages, such as the community health council, health authority or groups within the voluntary or independent sectors. This does not mean, though, that contact should be made with these groups, potentially raising expectations before discussing your plans within your organisation. However, having done this, it may be worthwhile eliciting a sounding from these groups about your hypotheses.

Project planning can be extremely helpful, if you have not already had to provide that level of information at an earlier stage. This does not have to be complicated: use your rich picture or relationship diagram as a basis. The key information you need in the plan are the resources required, the timescales, and the expected stages and outcomes. The other point to remember is that if any one of these changes part way through, it has a knock-on effect on the other two parts. For example, it is unlikely that, if the timescales are halved, you will be able to complete the project or certainly provide the level of detail originally agreed.

A simple Gantt chart (Fig. 9.7) is a useful *aide-mémoire* showing the days or dates across the top of the page and a list of tasks down the left-hand side. Keep the tasks in chronological order. You then draw a line across for each task showing the proposed start and finish date.

There is, of course, an element of frustration to be built into change of this sort. Managers may not be able to give you the support you feel you

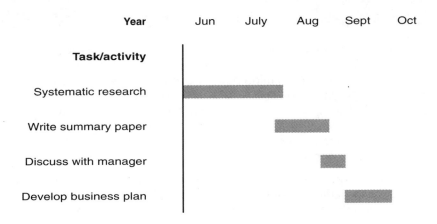

Figure 9.7 Example of a Gantt chart for project planning.

need, particularly with so many major changes taking place within the NHS at present. Colleagues may feel threatened or not understand the need to change (remember how important that felt-need is to models of change management). The structure and culture of the organisation may help or hinder. Highly centralised organisations may be very inflexible, but there may be someone who you can interest in this project who can facilitate key issues for you. Centralised training departments can make life easier as a wonderful resource for you to tap into.

Most of us have been guilty at some point in our careers of saying, 'I know what I should be doing . . . but it's not always possible because . . .' evidence-based practice is useful in many cases, but does have limitations, as the example below illustrates.

Evidence-based practice shows that graduated compression stockings can prevent postoperative venous thromboembolism in individuals who are at medium risk. It is less conclusive for those in the high-risk categories and, if the weather is very hot, individuals complain about how uncomfortable they are wearing them in the heat. What do you do as a practitioner?

It is also worth considering whether it is more appropriate to introduce the practice as a big bang or more softly softly, perhaps as a pilot scheme or phased implementation. The particular type of evidence-based practice you are introducing, together with consideration of the culture and structure of the organisation, will all be deciding factors. Remember as well that you are more likely to effect change within organisations that are flexible, working towards continuous improvement, and where you have senior management support.

How do your outcome measures relate to the research that the practice was originally based on?

From a management perspective this is a question you will undoubtably be asked, and hopefully have already asked yourself. Are there further improvements to be made? Can you match the results in the research? If not, what are the causal factors? Can these be altered or is it a case of managing around current immoveables (are they organisational immoveables or can a more senior manager effect change management?). Or have you surpassed the expected results?

Evaluation of evidence-based practice is essential and, if you think back to earlier in the chapter, a key part of change management to ensure that the changes have been in the right direction and producing the desired outcomes. That is not to say that you must adhere rigidly to an action plan, if there are improvements to be made or changing external situations that you must take into account.

To simplify greatly a hard systems approach: plan → do → review. Proof of lasting change for the better, and hopefully good news for all concerned, is necessary to justify the change in the first place: show improvements in care, allow individuals and their carers to see that they have an input and impact on the changed services. It is also important for your individual credibility within the organisation.

Feedback to all stakeholders is important. How often have we muttered about the informational Black Hole. Information is sucked in, never to be seen again. You can do this in a number of ways, such as a newsletter for regular updates or verbal reporting to small groups. As with other communication, think about the audience and target your message in terms of content and modality.

Key points

- There are three main stages that link with management of change: analysis and planning; implementation and action plan; evaluation and consolidation.
- At each stage think about the differing audience or stakeholders involved and how you need to adapt the content and modality of the message.
- Feedback at the evaluation stage is crucial for consolidation of the changes to and by the stakeholders.

FEATURES OF SUCCESSFUL ORGANISATIONS

We have described different structures and cultures of organisations. Some of you will find a fairly homogeneous pattern and will be able to identify your structure and culture easily. Others may recognise aspects from several of the models and will need to adopt a more eclectic approach. So far no judgements have been made on what is good or bad, but care has been taken to stress that the culture and structure depend very much on the business of the organisation.

Of the many theories on successful organisations available, some appear to have withstood the test of time better than others, which is why we make no apology for using the following example. Peters and Waterman (1982) identified eight main principles or attributes of excellence:

1. Action – the organisation is able to make a rapid and appropriate response
2. Close to the customer – the organisation learns from its clients
3. Autonomy and entrepreneurship – innovators and entrepreneurs are encouraged
4. Productivity through people – individuals and their contributions are respected
5. Hands on/value driven – organisational values are recognised throughout and managers 'walk the talk'

6. Stick to the knitting – work on what you know and in which you have the expertise
7. Simple form/lean staff – simple structure and lean levels of senior management
8. Simultaneous loose/tight properties – organisational culture and understanding of values allows tight control, whilst allowing individuals to be autonomous and innovative.

Good communication is essential to underpin the above and for any organisation to function successfully. Organisations that are constantly working to improve their services also tend to be more successful.

This chapter has concentrated on the application of evidence-based practice to clinical issues, within a management framework. It is worth reflecting that there is a growing recognition of evidence-based management. Research into management practice generally produces less clear evidence than in clinical research. This is at least partially due to the problems in identifying the key variables, much less controlling them, as is possible in some clinical research. However, from an organisational perspective, the features of organisations that support and encourage evidence-based practice are also those capable of promoting evidence-based management. They foster a learning or research culture, within which you can develop self-reflection and work continuously to improve your practice, be it clinical or management.

The process is also the same for evidence-based medicine, as Sackett (1997) has shown:

• converting information needs into answerable questions
• finding the 'best' evidence to answer those questions
• critically appraising the evidence for validity and applicability
• evaluating your own performance.

Remembering that evidence-based practice, medicine or management can inform, but does not replace, your own clinical or management expertise is perhaps the most important point.

WHAT TYPE OF ORGANISATION DO YOU WORK IN?

This section is intended to summarise in question format all the issues raised within the chapter and to encourage you to think about the dynamics of your organisation. As a result, you may wish to modify or try a different approach to that which you would normally adopt.

• You have already spent time earlier in the chapter assessing the different aspects of your organisational culture and structure. How do these link with the above attributes?
• Does the culture or structure enable or hamper the organisation in meeting its goals?

- Does it enable you and your department or division to meet your goals and therefore the organisational goals?
- What are the environmental factors influencing changes (policy, mergers, changes, etc.) – internal and external?
- Who are the change agents within your organisation?
- What awareness or importance is attached to evidence-based practice within your organisation?
- What examples are there already in practice?

CONCLUSIONS

Any healthcare organisation needs to be responsive and flexible to the changing needs of the environment. Analysis of the internal and external environment will afford you a greater understanding of the context in which the change is to take place. It also allows you an opportunity to assess whether now is the right time to broach change and how and who to approach.

Evidence-based practice is a useful tool to introduce, justify and evaluate change and changing practice within healthcare. It enables you to question whether there are more effective ways of achieving the same outcomes and whether there are improvements to existing outcomes that can be made. It is an important external driver for change from a national policy perspective and will underpin the need for clinical governance and accountability. Much very good work has already been produced either via research or audit projects in both acute and primary care sectors. Although the chapter concentrates primarily on using existing information, it also highlights the need to manage areas where there is little or no evidence available. The absence of evidence-based practice does not equate with no need for services currently provided. The rationale for providing or not providing healthcare services in this situation requires careful consideration. It also identifies areas that could benefit from research or audit projects.

You should remember that evidence-based practice is another tool to help along the 'rock-strewn pathway' and is not intended to be used in isolation and to the exclusion of other methods.

Key points

- Communicate: develop and use your networks.
- Broaden your outlook: from your current focal point, gain an understanding of the wider context.
- Opportunities: use and create them to influence at all levels
- Challenge assumptions and beliefs using evidence-based practice.
- Create a positive impact on the organisation and, more importantly, patient care.

REFERENCES

Bullock, R.J. & Batten, D. (1985). It's just a phase we're going through: a review and synthesis of organisational development (OD) phase analysis. *Group and Organisation Studies*, **10**, 383–412.

French, W.L. & Bell, C.H. (1984). *Organisation Development*. Engelwood Cliffs, New Jersey: Prentice Hall.

Porter O'Grady, T. (1995). *The Leadership Revolution in Health Care. Altering Systems, Changing Behaviours*. Gaithersburg, MD: Aspen.

Peters, T.J. & Waterman, R.H. (1982). *In Search of Excellence: Lessons from America's Best Run Companies*. London: Harper & Row.

Sackett, D.L. (1997). The need for evidence based medicine. In *Managing Medicine: A Survival Guide*, ed. Sanderson, D. & Brown, J., pp. 23–31. London: Financial Times Healthcare.

Schein, E.H. (1985). *Organisation, Culture and Leadership: A Dynamic View*. San Francisco: Jossey-Bass.

Further Reading

Baird, L.S., Post, J.E. & Mahon, J.F. (1990). *Management: Function and Responsibilities*. New York: HarperCollins.

Burnes, B. (1992). *Managing Change*. London: Pitman Publishing.

Checkland, P. (1981). *Systems Thinking, Systems Practice*. Chichester: Wiley.

Lessem, R. (1989). *Global Management Principles*. Hemel Hempstead: Prentice Hall International.

Moore, A., McQuay, H. & Gray, M. (1995). *Bandolier: the first 20, issues*. Oxford: Classic Press.

Øvretveit, J. (1998). Evidence-based management technologies in health care. *Healthcare Quality*, **4**(1), 21–25.

Porter O'Grady, T (1984). *Shared Governance for Nursing*. Gaithersburg, MD: Aspen.

Stewart, R. (1998). More art than science? *Health Service Journal*, **26 March**, pp. 28–29.

Thompson, J.L. (1990). *Strategic Management Awareness and Change*. London: Chapman & Hall.

Wilson, D.C. & Rosenfield, R.H. (1990). *Managing Organisations: Text, Readings and Cases*. London: McGraw-Hill.

10 Ethical change

Gill Collinson

KEY ISSUES

◆ Healthcare ethics

◆ Influence of personal and social values in evidence-based healthcare

◆ Allocation of healthcare resources

◆ Aspects of clinical governance, professional self-regulation, codes of practice and informed consent

◆ Strategies for ethical decision making in clinical practice

INTRODUCTION

The concept of evidence-based healthcare seeks to ensure that the services, procedures and practice of professionals offered to users and clients is, wherever possible, based on the best evidence that it will be of benefit. Evidence from research, audit, the opinion of experts and the views of users all contribute to decisions regarding the best way to provide healthcare across the spectrum of specialities, environments and contexts that make up health services. Central to this is whether a particular practice or procedure is clinically effective, and has been defined as 'doing the right thing, in the right way, and at the right time, for the right patient' (Royal College of Nursing, 1996). However, determining what is right for a population or an individual cannot be based only upon evidence of effectiveness derived by research. Personal and social values and beliefs, culture, past experience and individual choice also influence such decisions.

Introducing and managing change, whether at practice, organisational or policy level, has to take account of the evidence derived through systematic research-based enquiry and these other influencing factors.

This chapter seeks to introduce you to some of these factors and to illustrate how moral or ethical dimensions impact upon achieving evidence-based healthcare. By the end of this chapter you will be able to:

- define the term 'healthcare ethics'
- understand how personal and social values influence decision making
- identify levels and methods of healthcare resource allocation
- start to explore the ethical aspects of clinical governance
- identify and use strategies to recognise and support the ethical dimension of practice-based decisions.

WHAT ARE ETHICS?

The word ethics, derived from the Greek term *ethos,* originally meant conduct, customs and character. Morals, derived from the Latin *mores,* means custom or habit. We now use the term ethics or morals to describe a branch of philosophy that deals with questions of human conduct that are important to all individuals, groups and societies. Each society, religion and profession has principles or standards of conduct, which provide guidance to members. Healthcare ethics deals with the moral questions and issues raised within the healthcare context (Beauchamp and Childress, 1994). These range from the situations in the clinical setting, which focus on individual patients and their family, to those concerned with broader policy decisions relating to the allocation of resources. The decisions that are ultimately made in any given situation will be influenced strongly by personal or societal beliefs and values.

BELIEFS AND VALUES

Beliefs are firmly held opinions, which may or may not be true in reality. We acquire them through experience and they may be influenced by the attitudes and behaviours of others. For example, as children we may adopt many of our parents' beliefs, only to find they change as we experience the world independently.

In the course of their practice, healthcare professionals meet people whose beliefs are very different from their own. Practitioners have to adopt a non-judgemental attitude towards the beliefs of those they are caring for and ensure that they respect each individual's beliefs. Ethical dilemmas can occur for practitioners when patients' expressed beliefs are in conflict with the proposed course of treatment or care which is known through research-based evidence to offer the patient the best outcome.

The example below illustrates how difficult it can be for healthcare professionals always to respect individuals' beliefs. Uncomfortable feelings and emotions may be felt, despite knowing intellectually that respecting an individual's beliefs is the right course of action.

Example: Individual beliefs A young woman is admitted to the accident and emergency department following a road traffic accident. She has multiple injuries and requires surgery, which is likely to necessitate a blood transfusion. She is conscious and informs the staff that her religious beliefs are such that she will not consent to a blood transfusion. What do you think the staff should do? How do you think you would feel in this situation?

In the same way as each of us has our own personal beliefs, which may be different from those of others, beliefs differ between cultures and societies. For example, in the UK healthcare is funded mainly from taxation and is a public service, because generally British society believes that healthcare is a fundamental human right of all citizens, which should be available regardless of the ability to pay. By contrast, in the USA healthcare is predominantly funded by individuals, via insurance, because there is a fundamental belief that individuals have the right to choose how to spend their income and that the state should interfere as little as possible. These examples show how beliefs influence different societies and how subsequently whole systems of services are developed and delivered, such as health and social care, education and criminal justice.

Values are the social principles that give meaning and direction to individuals, groups and organisations. They influence behaviour and underpin the choices and decisions made in life, albeit often unconsciously. Observation of people's behaviour will often illustrate their values, yet many do not take the time to clarify their own values and as a result may find themselves in situations where they feel uncomfortable and at odds with others.

Raths, Harmin and Simon (1978) describe a process by which values can be determined or clarified. The process comprises three main categories, choosing, prizing and acting:

1. Choosing is the intellectual or cognitive aspect of valuing. Values are ideally chosen freely, having considered alternatives.
2. Prizing is the emotional or affective aspect. It is important to feel good about one's values.
3. Acting is the behavioural aspect. People affirm their values by making them part of their behaviour.

Reflection Make a list of the values you believe to be important to your profession, e.g. caring, equity, promotion of health, independence, etc. Using the process of valuing described above, think about each of the values you have listed and see which of these values are most important to you.

Each of us will have developed a different list of values that are important to us personally, but some values frequently cited and discussed by healthcare professionals are regarded as being particularly important. These include confidentiality, autonomy, informed consent and duty of care.

POLICY AND HEALTHCARE DELIVERY

Earlier chapters have discussed how increasingly over the past few decades the need and demand for healthcare has increased, due to four main factors. Muir Gray (1997) describes these factors as:

- an ageing population
- new technology and knowledge
- increased patient expectations
- increased professional expectations.

However, growth in the available resources for healthcare has not risen at the same rate as the increase in demand. As a result there has been increasing pressure on healthcare organisations and professionals to demonstrate that services, procedures and practice are both clinically and cost effective (see Chapters 1 and 5).

Evidence-based healthcare is therefore an important strand in the strategy for ensuring that the available resources are allocated effectively and the services provided are of high quality. Individually or collectively healthcare professionals are involved in the development and implementation of policy. Davis and Aroskar (1991, p. 213) define policy as 'a course of action or inaction selected from among alternatives in the context of given conditions to guide present and future decisions and implementation of those decisions'. Healthcare policy can therefore be seen as a framework for guiding decisions, made by individuals, groups or organisations, responsible for commissioning or providing healthcare services. Policy at all levels is underpinned by values and should be informed by evidence.

Research-based evidence assists decisions to be made at a number of levels including those made by:

- individual clinicians
- a group or team
- department or directorate
- healthcare provider organisation (NHS Trust, general practice, nursing home)
- healthcare commissioning agency (Health Authority or Primary Care Group)
- government.

ALLOCATION OF RESOURCES

The basic economic problem facing healthcare systems around the world, including the NHS, is how to control costs and to distribute resources efficiently and effectively in order to satisfy human needs and desires. In contrast, the basic ethical problem is how to structure a healthcare system that fairly distributes resources and provides equitable access to health services at a manageable cost. These economic and ethical problems are closely intertwined and may manifest as conflict or dilemmas in the formation of healthcare policy. The most sensitive of these dilemmas is what we have come to know as rationing.

Rationing is not a popular phrase and Klein (1992) argues that 'it is invoked to make the flesh creep' rather than 'to prompt argument about how best to deal with the inescapable'. What is clear from the literature is that different commentators interpret rationing in different ways.

The main distinction appears to be in whether rationing is about withholding resources in the form of treatment and care or determining the best way to use available resources (Royal College of Physicians, 1995). Those who propose the latter interpretation often refer to priority setting rather than rationing, although these terms are used interchangeably by many writers.

What is clear in all definitions is that the elimination of care that provides no benefits at all does not constitute rationing. Evidence that shows treatments to be ineffective is clearly as important as evidence that shows effectiveness. However, convincing some practitioners that this is so may be difficult if they *believe* as a result of their experience that a particular practice is effective.

Reflection   Can you think of an example from your own sphere of practice, where evidence has shown something to be ineffective, but it has been difficult to convince your colleagues that this is so?

Changing someone's beliefs can be very difficult, which is why having robust evidence is only part of the jigsaw when you are endeavouring to implement evidence-based practice and to change behaviour, as discussed in previous chapters.

Macro, medium and micro

The allocation of resources is often categorised as macro, medium and micro. The first dimension, macro, is deciding how much to allocate to healthcare as against competing demands on public resources, such as education, housing and defence. These decisions are made by government, society's elected representatives, and the priority they give to any particular area of public spending will in part reflect the values and beliefs of the political party in power. There will always be much discussion and debate regarding how much of the public purse should be allocated to any particular area of expenditure. This, however, does not eliminate the need to consider how the resources available to healthcare should be best allocated.

This dimension – medium-level allocation – is where decisions regarding which treatments or services have priority are made and is the area where much of the current debate centres. Responsibility for such decisions within the NHS lies with commissioners of healthcare, usually district health authorities, although there are a range of models of commissioning, the most recent being primary care groups (Department of Health, 1997). Having been tasked to find socially acceptable and justifiable criteria on which to allocate resources, those responsible for such decisions around the globe have taken a variety of approaches.

In some countries, such as the USA and the Netherlands, there have been proposals for limiting the conditions or treatments paid for by the state to those that are considered, after public consultation, to have priority (Brannigan, 1995). The best known of these initiatives is what has come to be known as the Oregon Experiment (see Case study).

Other countries, such as New Zealand, have rejected the concept that a patient's need can necessarily be assessed by the type of diagnosis and have concentrated instead on strategies that maximize the effectiveness of treatment – what we have come to call evidence-based healthcare. Chapter 5 discusses some of the methods available to healthcare commissioners and providers to develop clinically effective services and positive outcomes.

The third dimension of rationing, often referred to as micro allocation, is that which takes place at the patient–professional interface. It is at this level that the common forms of prioritising patients occur, such as the use of waiting lists. Here doctors and other healthcare professionals choose how to use the resources available to them, generally on the basis of need. For example, patients with a life-threatening condition will generally be given higher priority than those with non-life-threatening conditions.

Case study: The Oregon Experiment The development of the Oregon plan began in the 1980s when the US State of Oregon took steps to confront difficulties with the allocation of Medicaid funds, the public assistance programme for the poor. An estimated 400, 000 Oregonians had no health insurance, and of these 280, 000 were from from working households and therefore did not qualify to receive Medicaid. Indeed, if a family earned more than US$6960 per year they were not eligible for state assistance.

Following the Governors Conference on Health Care for the Medically Poor in 1982, Oregon Health Decisions Incorporated (OHD) was established. OHD held over 300 public meetings, involving

Case study cont'd

over 5000 citizens, with the aim of raising awareness regarding the allocation of Medicaid resources.

Over the years the plan has been further developed and refined so that health services available through Medicaid are prioritised, by a process of public participation and cost–utility analysis. The available resources are then determined and the services of high priority are funded and those of lower priority are not. The plan was finally approved by the Secretary of Health and Human Services, with the uninsured being phased into the scheme over a 5-year period.

Obtaining and appraising the values of the citizens of Oregon was a fundamental strand of the plan's development. In addition to public meetings, telephone surveys were conducted and testimonies from a variety of interest groups were heard.

The five values of most concern were prevention, equity, quality of life, the ability to function and cost effectiveness. However, the demographic data of those attending meetings shows us just how difficult it can be to obtain a representative sample of public opinion.

Of those attending meetings, 69% were healthcare workers. Those who would be the first to be affected by the plan (i.e. low-income groups) were critically underrepresented. In addition, experience of a specific problem appeared to play an important role in how it was perceived. Those with experience perceived a particular condition to be less serious than those with no experience of the condition.

Source: Oregon Health Services Commission (1991).

Waiting lists

Waiting lists for inpatient treatment are a major issue in the NHS and the focus of considerable concern by all political parties. In recent years there have been an increasing number of government initiatives to reduce both waiting lists and waiting times.

Waiting lists are confined almost exclusively to elective non-urgent treatment, with patients requiring emergency care being treated immediately. The reasons why waiting lists exist is not entirely clear, but the theory that they arise simply because demand exceeds supply is the most common and intuitively appealing (Harvey, 1993). However, if demand permanently exceeded supply, waiting lists would extend into infinity and, whilst there has been some overall increase in recent years, many waiting lists appear to stabilize at a particular length.

Supporters of the view that waiting lists are merely a backlog of cases accumulated over time argue that they can be cleared by a temporary increase in treatment rates. The initiatives of the past few years have test-ed this theory: extra resources have been made available to clear patients who have been on the list longest. Such initiatives have also raised ethical concerns regarding whether it is justifiable to treat those who have waited a long time in preference to those who have an urgent need for treatment.

Despite the fact that waiting lists are generally unpopular and regarded as a bad thing, they may be considered to have some benefits. Higgins and Ruddle (1991) argue that although 'it is easy to criticise waiting lists and queues as methods of rationing scarce NHS resources . . . the alternatives may be worse'. The main alternative would be to exclude some forms of treatment that are currently available. Those in favour of exclusion argue that it is more honest to refuse access to waiting lists than to leave people on them for years, whereas the contrary argument is that being on a waiting list at least offers them some hope. It is interesting to note that, as the resource allocation debate has developed, some of those initially in favour of introducing explicit forms of rationing are, as a result of the difficulties associated with them, beginning to once again look more favourably towards waiting lists (Klein, 1992).

Age

A further criterion utilised in resource allocation decisions is age, which has been used to make decisions such as those regarding which patients are eligible for haemodialysis and transplantation (Kilner, 1990). Discriminating against older people in this way has, however, been con-demned by the Royal College of Physicians (1994) and the Medical Research Council (1994) as being inequitable and lacking justification. Despite this condemnation, arguments have been made to support age as a criterion for resource allocation in healthcare, namely the 'fair innings argument'. Harris (1988, p. 119) describes this view as concentrating 'on the idea that it cannot be just that someone who has already had more than his fair share of life and its delights should be preferred to the younger per-son who has not been so favoured'. Therefore it is argued that society is likely to benefit more if a younger person is saved in preference to an older person. In contrast to this view is the 'just rewards' argument, that age dis-crimination is not just because of the past contributions made to society, or more specifically to the NHS, by the elderly (Hunter and Harrison, 1994).

The use of age as a patient selection device is most often linked with other criteria, rather than used overtly. Some argue, for example, that using age is legitimate because it screens out the elderly, who are less likely to benefit from some forms of treatment and have poorer outcomes. Against this Grimley Evans (1991) claims that there is a persistent misunderstand-ing of the link between age and the ability to benefit from high technology medicine and that, if an age criterion is used, it should be physiological rather than chronological.

As the proportion of elderly persons in the population rises and their need for personal care as well as medical care increases, resource allocation decisions will often focus on this group. The fact that they are often vulnerable means that they may provide little resistance to decisions that discriminate against them, which some would argue would make them a special case (Kilner, 1990).

Some surveys have, however, shown that the public supports the use of age as a criterion for patient selection, specifically that resources should be directed to the young rather than the old, and if public participation in resource allocation decisions increases, as advocated by current policy, it is possible that the use of old age as a rationing device may become more prevalent and socially, if not morally, acceptable (Jennings, 1993).

So far in this chapter I have described some of the most commonly debated formal methods and criteria used in allocating healthcare resources. However, healthcare professionals make decisions everyday about how they will prioritise their workload, which directly affects patients. We often make these decisions automatically; for example, which patient will we see first, the patient just back from the operating theatre or the patient waiting to go home who needs some instruction on when to take their medication? Or who needs more of our time, the bereaved relative or the confused woman who needs help to eat her supper? Generally we just get on with what needs to be done, but there are days when we might finish work and realise that we feel uncomfortable because we have had to compromise to much. This may be the spur to consciously reflect on events, clarify our values and start to explore how we make these decisions and whether changing our practice in some way might improve the situation.

Reflection   Take some time to reflect on a recent day at work:

- What did you do and in what sequence?
- How did you prioritise what needed to be done?
- Were you able to be proactive and plan your activities or were you in a position of responding to the requests and demands of others?
- How did it make you feel?
- What are the characteristics of a day at work when you feel fulfilled?
- What are the characteristics of a day at work when you feel frustrated?
- Can you identify a link between these characteristics and the values you identified as being important to you as a healthcare professional earlier in the chapter?

I hope that this reflective activity has illustrated to you the importance of values and ethics in clinical decision making. As Levine (1990, p. 41) has written:

There are overlooked ethical challenges in the mundane everyday activities of professional practice and these have gone largely unexamined. Ethical behaviour is not the display of one's moral rectitude in times of crisis. It is the day-by-day expression of one's commitment to other persons and the ways in which human beings relate to one another in their daily interactions.

ASPECTS OF CLINICAL GOVERNANCE

The recent consultation document *A First Class Service* (Department of Health, 1998) outlines this government's proposals for improving the quality of care and services in the NHS. This strategy builds on many of the aspects of improving healthcare already discussed in this book, including improving the evidence base, implementing the evidence and monitoring standards. Research and development, clinical effectiveness initiatives such as guidelines and national service frameworks, audit and practice development are all part of what has been named clinical governance. In addition, local NHS organisations will be required to take on responsibility for all aspects of clinical governance and will be accountable for making sure standards are met. Chief executives of NHS Trusts will be accountable for the standards of care within an organisation, as individual practitioners are accountable for their practice.

This organisational responsibility does not negate individuals from taking responsibility, but requires organisations to ensure that systems and processes are in place to ensure that standards are maintained. Practitioners and managers in organisations will need to work in partnership. For example, all practitioners will need to maintain and update their professional skills and knowledge. Individuals must be motivated to learn and take responsibility for their ongoing professional development. At the same time organisations will be required to support lifelong learning and put systems in place to enable practitioners to maintain their competence.

A further element of clinical governance is ensuring that standards of professional self-regulation are rigorous, that the standards of professional conduct are such that they protect the public and meet the valid expectations of patients and society in general. As professional self-regulation encompasses important aspects of human conduct or ethics, and is an essential part of providing quality care, this will be discussed further in this chapter.

PROFESSIONAL SELF-REGULATION

Professional self-regulation allows health professions to set their own standards of professional practice, conduct and discipline. The role of professional regulatory bodies such as the General Medical Council (GMC), the UK Central Council for Nursing, Midwifery and Health Visiting (UKCC) and the Council for Professions Supplementary to Medicine is to set these standards and ensure that they keep pace with changes in clinical practice and expectations placed on healthcare professionals. To maintain the trust of the public at large, the professions must be openly accountable for the standards they set and the way these are enforced.

These standards are generally documented in a profession's code of practice or conduct, which provides guidelines and requirements that all members of the profession are expected to follow. Characteristically codes of practice gives guidance, in the form of principles regarding issues such as consent, confidentiality, autonomy, advocacy and duty of care. However, codes cannot deal with every conflict a registered practitioner may encounter. In some cases a choice of priorities has to be made and, as has been observed since Aristotle, judgement must be used in making decisions (Jackson, 1994). Accountability is about answering for your actions, being able to use your professional knowledge, skills and judgement to make a decision, and being able to account for your decision. Evidence, in the many forms discussed in this book, is therefore crucial to all practitioners being able to exercise accountability.

It is not the purpose of this chapter to discuss ethical theories and issues in detail; however, of the principles outlined in professional codes, one of the most significant in terms of evidence-based practice is that of informed consent. I shall therefore use it to illustrate how evidence-based practice is not the same as research-based practice, although the terms are often used interchangeably, and that providing high-quality clinical care is a complex phenonomen.

INFORMED CONSENT

The issue of consent has been widely discussed, debated and developed ever since the Nuremburg trials which brought to the world's attention horrifying evidence of medical experimentation in concentration camps. As the concept of informed consent developed, it has seen a shift from the practitioner's obligation to disclose information towards the quality of a patient's understanding and consent.

Nearly all professional codes hold that healthcare practitioners must obtain the informed consent of patients before treatment or care, and procedures for consent should be designed to enable patients to make an autonomous choice. It is essential that practitioners give patients adequate information, in a manner that is sensitive and enables understanding. Time is essential for patients to consider proposed courses of action and they may wish to discuss their options with others. Informed consent is not just about those occasions when written consent is required, for example before surgery. Patients can demonstrate their decision in a number of ways including verbally or by cooperating. They may also withdraw their consent in the same ways.

As evidence-based practice has developed, the related concept of evidence-based choice has developed, which will inevitably impact on the way informed consent is obtained. Muir Gray (1997) suggests that, when appraising the best available evidence to provide patients with evidence-based information, the practitioner should calculate:

- the probability that the patient will benefit
- the magnitude of any benefit
- the probability that the patient will suffer adverse effects of treatment
- the magnitude of any adverse effects.

Written information, in the form of patient leaflets, should ideally include the strength of the evidence supporting it, such as the patient information booklets produced by the Agency for Health Care Policy and Research discussed in Chapter 5.

Some practitioners may argue that it is difficult to produce evidence-based information in a way that patients can easily understand but research has shown that the provision of evidence does alter patients' views and decisions. For example, in a study by Murphy *et al.* (1994) people aged between 60 and 99 years were asked whether they wished to receive cardiopulmonary resuscitation. Initially 41% agreed that they would; however, after being given information regarding the evidence in relation to likely survival, the proportion still wishing to receive it fell to 22%. Clearly then, evidence is important not only to the decisions made by healthcare professionals, but also to those made by patients. As the amount of evidence increases and its quality improves, practitioners will have an obligation not only to ensure they incorporate it into their practice, but that they make this information available to patients to enable them to make autonomous choices based on sound evidence.

Reflection Think about the information you regularly give to the patients you care for. Do you incorporate research-based information? Does the written information you give to patients refer to research-based evidence? Does the information you provide allow patients to make informed decisions? Can you think of ways that you and your colleagues can improve the quality of information you provide?

STRATEGIES FOR SUPPORTING ETHICAL DECISION MAKING

As illustrated in the previous section, most professions are provided with guidance regarding ethical issues in the form of their professional code of practice. Codes are both a public statement of professional standards and provide practitioners with guidance regarding what is expected of them in the course of their practice. They are, however, unable to provide practitioners with support regarding specific cases (Beyerstein, 1993).

In the UK the only formal means of considering ethical issues are local research ethics committees, which meet to consider the ethical issues relating to proposed research activity. Local research ethics committees must be consulted regarding any research proposal involving:

- NHS patients
- fetal material and in vitro fertilisation involving NHS patients
- the recently dead, in NHS premises
- access to the records of past or present NHS patients
- the use of, or potential access to, NHS premises or facilities.

You can obtain further information regarding the procedures of your local research ethics committee from the district health authority or lead person for research and development in your organisation. There are, however, no formal mechanisms to support practitioners regarding ethical issues that arise in daily practice in this country. This is not the case in other parts of the world, in particular the USA, where an increasing range of mechanisms is being developed to support practitioners. These include:

- ethics committees
- ethics rounds
- ethics consultation services.

Ethics committees

There has been a remarkable growth in the number of US healthcare institutions establishing ethics committees over the past two decades, from less than 1% of hospitals in 1982 to approximately 60% in 1988 (Hoffman, 1993). The motivation for establishing these committees has been both internal, intitiated by healthcare professionals looking for a better way to deal with clinical ethical issues, and by influential external events.

Amongst these external influences was the 1976 New Jersey court case of Karen Ann Quinlan, a young woman in a persistent vegetative state, whose father requested the legal right to authorise her removal from a ventilator. In giving its opinion the New Jersey Supreme Court quoted an article by Dr Karen Teel (1975) which suggested that the way to improve decision making in such cases would be for hospitals to establish ethics committees.

These committees are generally multidisciplinary and serve a number of functions including:

- reviewing ethical and others values involved in patient care
- making broader ethical and policy decisions
- providing support for healthcare professionals involved in decisions of an ethical nature
- reviewing individual cases (Veatch, 1977).

Unfortunately there appears to be little evidence regarding the effectiveness of these committees and their success depends largely on the strengths of the chairperson and how seriously committee members and the organisation believe in its function (Davis and Aroskar, 1991).

Ethics rounds

Ethics rounds are similar to other nursing or medical rounds, except that the focus is on the ethical rather than the clinical perspectives of an individual case. At the University of California in San Francisco, ethics rounds were first established in neonatology and are conducted rather like a ward round in the UK, although there is a variety of formats that can be adopted (Glover, Ozar and Thomasana, 1986). The more typical type of ethics round seen in the USA is based on the format of the Grand Round, a presentation of one or more similar cases by one person, which is then discussed by a larger audience. This method works most effectively when teaching large numbers of students. It does have limitations in that it reduces very complex situations to one perspective, namely that of the person presenting the case (Andereck, 1992).

Ethical consultation services

An increasingly popular method of providing support to healthcare professionals facing difficult ethical issues is the provision of ethical consultation services. These work on a number of levels and provide a range of functions including consultation on difficult cases, suggestions for policy development, teaching and research (Thomasana, 1992). The service may be formal or informal, integral to the work of the ethics committee, or a separate service. They are the most recent development in the USA and appear to be flourishing at a time when the healthcare system is in crisis and faces innumerable ethical problems arising from advances in healthcare technology and inequity in the availability of services.

A model for ethical decision making

Although there may be a dearth of formal mechanisms specifically for considering ethical issues in the UK, practitioners can individually or collectively consider these issues in forums such as clinical supervision, peer support groups, etc. Thompson and Thompson (1985, p. 99) have developed the following ten-step approach to ethical decision making:

1. Review the situation to determine health problems, key individuals, the ethical components and what decisions are required.
2. Gather any additional information.
3. Identify the ethical issues in the situation.
4. Identify personal and professional values.
5. Identify the values of key individuals.
6. Identify any existing conflicts in values.
7. Determine who should decide.
8. Identify the range of actions and anticipated outcomes.

9. Decide on a course of action and carry it out.
10. Evaluate the results.

Does this model seem familiar in some ways? It is not dissimilar to either the audit cycle or the nursing process. It focuses on the particular requirements such as values, but it essentially gathers evidence, interprets it, decides on a course of action and then evaluates the outcome.

Using the Thompson and Thompson (1985) model, consider the following case study.

Case study: Mr Brown   Mr Brown is a 75-year-old man who has carcinoma of the bronchus. He has been in and out of hospital for palliative treatment and care for the last 6 months. He is aware of his diagnosis and poor prognosis. He has told the nursing staff on numerous occasions that his only real enjoyment now is being able to have a cigarette. He knows that smoking is the likely cause of his cancer and that it probably aggravates his symptoms.

Mr Brown is admitted to hospital; his condition having deteriorated considerably, he is unable to walk unaided and has lost a lot of weight. He asks the nurse to help him to the smoking room on the ward so that he can enjoy a cigarette. However, since his last admission the hospital has introduced a total no-smoking policy.

How did you get on? Difficult, isn't it ? You know the research evidence and so does the patient. The values of the organisation are in conflict with the personal values of the patient, so finding a solution to the problem will be difficult. However, this is the type of situation that occurs daily in our practice. Whilst it may not get easier to make the decision, understanding the component parts can at least help you to be aware of why they are difficult.

CONCLUSIONS

Evidence-based practice has a lot to offer healthcare professionals, patients and organisations. However, achieving it is a complex and sometimes difficult task as a range of influences, not least values and beliefs, affect this process, whether you are making decisions regarding an individual patient, a service, or policy for the entire NHS.

REFERENCES

Andereck, W.S. (1992). Development of a hospital ethics committee. Lessons from five years of case consultations. *Cambridge Quarterly of Healthcare Ethics*, **1**(1), 41–50.
Beauchamp, T.L. & Childress, J.F. (1994). *Principles of Biomedical Ethics*, 4th edn. New York: Oxford University Press.

Beyerstein, D. (1993). The functions and limitations of professional codes of ethics. In *Applied Ethics*, ed. Winkler, E.R. & Coombs, J.R. pp. 416–425. London: Blackwells.

Brannigan M (1995). Oregon's experiment. In *Reforming Health Care: The Philosophy and Practice of International Health Reform*, ed. Seedhouse, D. pp. 27–52. Chichester, New York: John Wiley.

Davis, A. & Aroskar, M.A. (eds) (1991). *Ethical Dilemmas and Nursing Practice*, 3rd edn. Norwalk, Connecticut: Appleton & Lange.

Department of Health (1997). *The New NHS, Modern, Dependable*, London: HMSO.

Department of Health (1998). *A First Class Service, Quality in the NHS*, London: Department of Health.

Glover, J.J., Ozar, D.T. & Thomasana, D.C.S. (1986). Teaching ethics on rounds, the ethicist as teacher, consultant and decision maker. *Theological Medicine*, **July**, 13–32.

Grimley Evans, J. (1991). Ageing and rationing: physiology not age should determine care. *British Medical Journal*, **303**, 869–870.

Harris, J. (1988). EQALYTY. In *Health, Rights and Resources*, ed. Byrne, P., pp. 100–127. London: King Edwards Hospital Fund.

Harvey, I. (1993). And so to bed; access to inpatient services. In *Rationing and Rationality: The Persistence of Waiting Lists*, eds. Frankel, S.J. & West, R.R. London: Macmillan.

Higgins, J. & Ruddle, S. (1991). Waiting for a better alternative. *Health Services Journal*, **101**, 18–19.

Hoffman, D. (1993). Evaluating ethics committees; a view from the outside. *Millbank Quarterly*, **71**(4), 677–701.

Hunter, D. & Harrison, S. (1994). *Rationing Public Health Care*. London: Institute for Public Policy Research.

Jackson, J. (1994). Common codes: divergent practices. In *Ethics and the Professions*, ed. Chadwick, R. Aldershot: Avebury.

Jennings, K. (1993). Rationing and older people. *Critical Public Health*, **4**, 33–35.

Kilner, L.F. (1990). *Who Lives? Who Dies? Ethical Criteria in Patient Selection*. New Haven, Connecticut: Yale University Press.

Klein, R. (1992). Dilemmas and decisions. *Health Management Quarterly*, 2nd Quarter, 2.

Levine, M. (1990). Nursing ethics and the ethical nurse. In *Professional Ethics in Nursing*, ed. Thompson, J. & Thompson, H. pp. 39–46. Malabor, Florida: Krieger.

Medical Research Council (1994). *The Health of the UK's Elderly People*. London: MRC.

Muir Gray, J.A. (1997). *Evidence-based Healthcare: How to Make Health Policy and Management Decisions*. London: Churchill Livingstone.

Murphy, D.J., Burrows, D., Santilli, S. *et al.* (1994). The influence of the probability of survival on patients' preferences regarding cardiopulmonary resuscitation. *New England Journal of Medicine*, **330**, 565–569.

Oregon Health Services Commission (1991). *Prioritization of Health Services: A Report to the Governor and Legislature*. Portland, Oregon: Oregon Health Services Commission.

Raths, L. Harmin, M. & Simon, S. (1978). *Values and Teaching*, 2nd edn. Columbus, Ohio: Charles Merrill.

Royal College of Nursing (1996). *Clinical Effectiveness. A Royal College of Nursing Guide*. London: RCN.

Royal College of Physicians (1994). *Ensuring Equity and Quality of Care for Elderly People: The Interface between Geriatric Medicine and General (Internal) Medicine*. London: RCP.

Royal College of Physicians (1995). *Setting Priorities in the NHS*. London: RCP.

Teel, K. (1975). The physician's dilemma, a doctor's view. what should the law be? *Baylor Law Review*, **27**(6), 9.

Thomasana, D.C. (1992). Ethics consults at a university medical center. *Cambridge Quarterly of Health Care Ethics*, **1**(3), 217.

Thompson, J.B. & Thompson, H.O. (1985). *Bioethical Decision Making for Nurses*. Norwalk, Connecticut: Appleton-Century-Crofts.

Veatch, R.M. (1977). What is the scope of hospital ethics committees? *Hospital Medical Staff*, **6**(9), 24–30.

Appendix I
Research and development centres

Centre for Evidence Based Medicine (CEBM)
University Of Oxford
Nuffield Department of Clinical Medicine
Level 5
The Oxford Radcliffe NHS Trust
Headley Way
Headington
Oxford
OX3 9DV

Tel   0186 522 2941
Fax 0186 522 2901

E-mail olive@cebm.jr2.ox.ac
http://cebm.jr2.ox.ac.uk

Centre for Evidence Based Nursing
University of York
Information Service
Heslington
York
YO1 5DD

Tel   0190 443 4101
Fax 0190 443 4102

http://www.york.ac.uk/deps/hstd
/centres/evidence/ev-intro.htm

Department of Health R & D Directorate
NHS Executive Headquarters
Quarry House
Quarry Hill
Leeds
LS2 7UE

Tel   0113 254 6183
Fax 0113 254 6174

http://www.open.gov.uk/doh/
rdd1.htm

National Centre for Clinical Audit
BMA House
Tavistock Square
London
WC1H 9JP

Tel   0171 383 6451
Fax 0171 730 0194

NHS Centre for Reviews and Dissemination (CRD)
University of York
Information Service
Heslington
York
YO1 5DD

Tel   0190 443 3707
Fax 0190 443 3661

E-mail revdis@york.ac.uk
http://www.york.ac.uk/inst/crd/welcome.htm

UK Cochrane Centre
Summertown Pavilion
Middle Way
Oxford
OX2 7LG

Tel   0186 551 6300
Fax 0186 561 5311

http://www.cochrane.co.uk

UK Clearing House for Information on the Assessment of Health Outcomes
Nuffield Institute for Health
71–75 Clarendon Road
Leeds
LS2 9PL

Tel   0113 233 3940
Fax 0113 246 0899

http://www.leeds.ac.uk/nuffield/infoservices/ukch/home.html

The Joanna Briggs Institute for Evidence Based Nursing and Midwifery
Royal Adelaide Hospital
South Terrace
Adelaide
South Australia 5000

http://www.joannabriggs.edu.au

Index

Index